SCAN
for
Animated Audio eBook,
Vocabulary Cards,
Comprehension Questions,
Coloring Pages,
and more

MEET OUR CHARACTERS THROUGHOUT OUR SERIES!

Petra

Polo

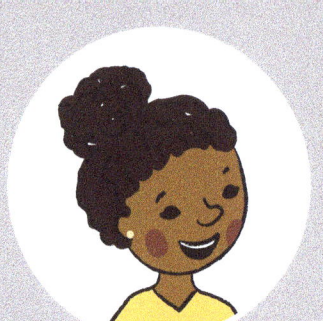
Lili

Dani

¡CONOCE A NUESTROS PERSONAJES A TRAVÉS DE NUESTRA SERIE!

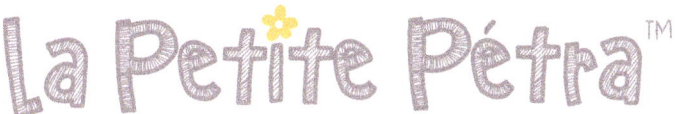

BILINGUAL PROGRAMS
FOR KIDS

PROGRAMAS BILINGÜES
PARA NIÑOS

18 TITLES
12 SERIES
5 LANGUAGES
Customized languages available on Special Orders

18 TÍTULOS
12 SERIES
5 IDIOMAS
Idiomas personalizados disponibles a través de pedidos especiales

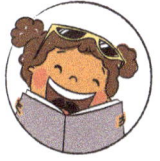

PHYSICAL BOOKS

ANIMATED AUDIO EBOOKS

VOCABULARY FLASHCARDS

COMPREHENSION QUESTIONS

COLORING SHEETS

PUZZLES GAMES

LIBRO EN PAPEL

AUDIOLIBRO ANIMADO

FICHAS DE VOCABULARIO

PREGUNTAS DE COMPRENSIÓN

PÁGINAS PARA COLOREAR

PUZZLES JUEGOS

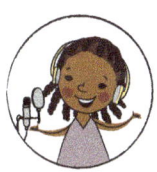
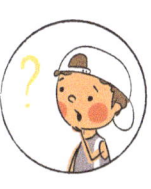
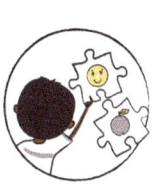
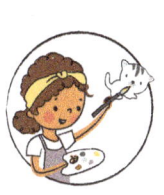

DEAR PARENTS AND TEACHERS,

Congratulations on encouraging your children and students to become bilingual and bilingually literate!

It is a decision that will pay dividends to your child or student for many years to come! Research has shown that it is easier for children who learn a language before the age of 6 to adopt a native accent. Research also shows that bilingual children have increased cognitive capacities.

The goal of Young and Bilingual™ is to accompany you and your children or students through the wonderful journey of becoming fully bilingual at a young age. The illustrations in each book are beautiful and colorful. Each book includes vocabulary words, a list of sight words used in the book, and phonics tips.

We have defined four different levels for our book series:

❶ Preschool-Kindergarten
Basic concepts and interactive reading for pre-readers

❷ Preschool to Grade 1
Simple sentences ideal for pre-readers, who are starting to learn how to read (under 150 words)

❸ Kindergarten to Grade 1
Short story ideal for beginner independent readers (under 300 words)

❹ Kindergarten to Grade 3
Short story, which includes life lessons and cultural discoveries (under 600 words)

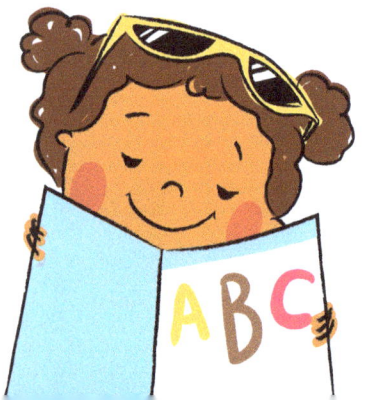

Young and Bilingual™ offers FREE supporting bilingual material on its website www.lapetitepetra.com to assist you and your children and students on this great journey of bilingualism. We welcome your feedback to improve continuously. Stay in touch with us, and, most importantly, enjoy the journey!

QUERIDOS PADRES Y PROFESORES,

¡Felicitaciones por animar a tus hijos y estudiantes a ser bilingües y a aprender a leer y escribir en varios idiomas!

¡Es una decisión que dará sus frutos en la vida de tu hijo o estudiante durante los años venideros! Los estudios demuestran que es más fácil tener un acento nativo si se aprende un idioma antes de los 6 años. Las investigaciones también han demostrado que los niños bilingües tienen mejores capacidades cognitivas.

El objetivo de Young and Bilingual™ es acompañarte a ti y a tus hijos o estudiantes en el maravilloso viaje de llegar a ser totalmente bilingües a una edad temprana. Las ilustraciones de todos los libros son hermosas y coloridas. Todos los libros incluyen palabras de vocabulario, una lista de palabras claves utilizadas en el libro y consejos de fonética.

Hemos definido cuatro niveles para nuestros libros:

❶ Preescolar-Jardín de Infancia
Conceptos básicos y lectura interactiva para pre-lectores

❷ Preescolar a Primer Grado
Frases sencillas ideales para pre-lectores que están empezando a aprender a leer (menos de 150 palabras)

❸ Jardín de Infancia a Primer Grado
Una historia corta, ideal para lectores autónomos principiantes (menos de 300 palabras)

❹ Jardín de Infancia a Tercer Grado
Una historia corta que incluye lecciones vitales y descubrimientos culturales (menos de 600 palabras)

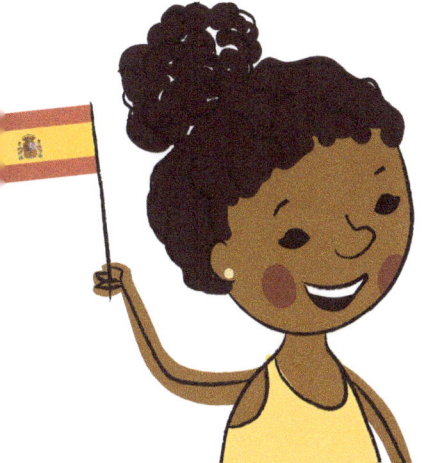

Young and Bilingual™ ofrece material de apoyo bilingüe GRATUITO en su sitio web www.lapetitepetra.com para ayudarte a ti y a tus hijos y estudiantes en este increíble viaje del bilingüismo. Agradecemos tus comentarios para mejorar continuamente. Manténte en contacto con nosotros y, sobre todo, ¡disfruta del viaje!

Publisher's Cataloging-In-Publication Data
(Prepared by Xponential Learning, Inc.)
Names: Krystel, Armand, author. | Vynokurova, Oksana, illustrator.
Title: Tus emociones son normales = Your emotions are normal / Krystel Armand ; illustrated by Oksana Vynokurova.
Other Titles: Tus emociones son normales / Your emotions are normal
Description: [Miami, Florida] : Xponential Learning Inc, 2020. | Series: La Petite Pétra | Bilingual. Spanish and English. | Interest age level: 005-010. | Summary: 'Emotions are normal but children must learn to manage their emotions to avoid getting overwhelmed. As parents, it is important for us to teach our children to recognize their feelings and learn to express them in a healthy way.'--Provided by publisher.

First Publication: May 2020
Third Edition May 2022
XPONENTIAL LEARNING INC
Copyright © 2020 Krystel Armand

All rights reserved. No part of this publication may be reproduced, distributed, or transmitted in any form or by any means, including photocopying, recording, or other electronic or mechanical methods, without the prior written permission of the publisher, except in the case of brief quotations embodied in critical reviews and certain other noncommercial uses permitted by copyright law.

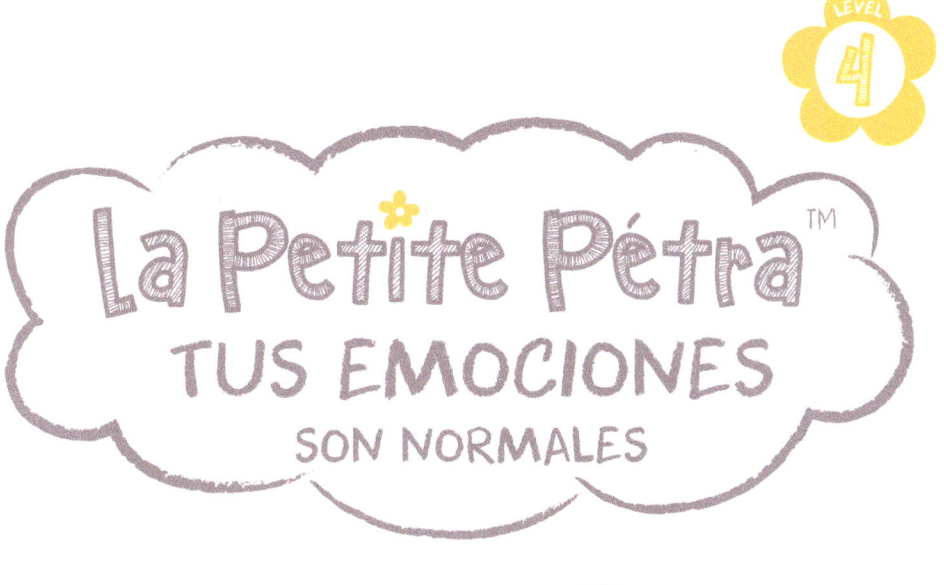

La Petite Pétra™
TUS EMOCIONES
SON NORMALES

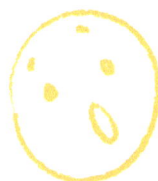
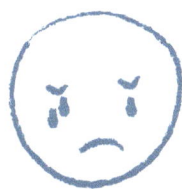

Your emotions are normal

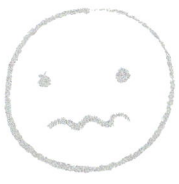

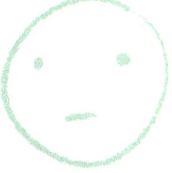

Krystel Armand
Illustrated by Oksana Vynokurova

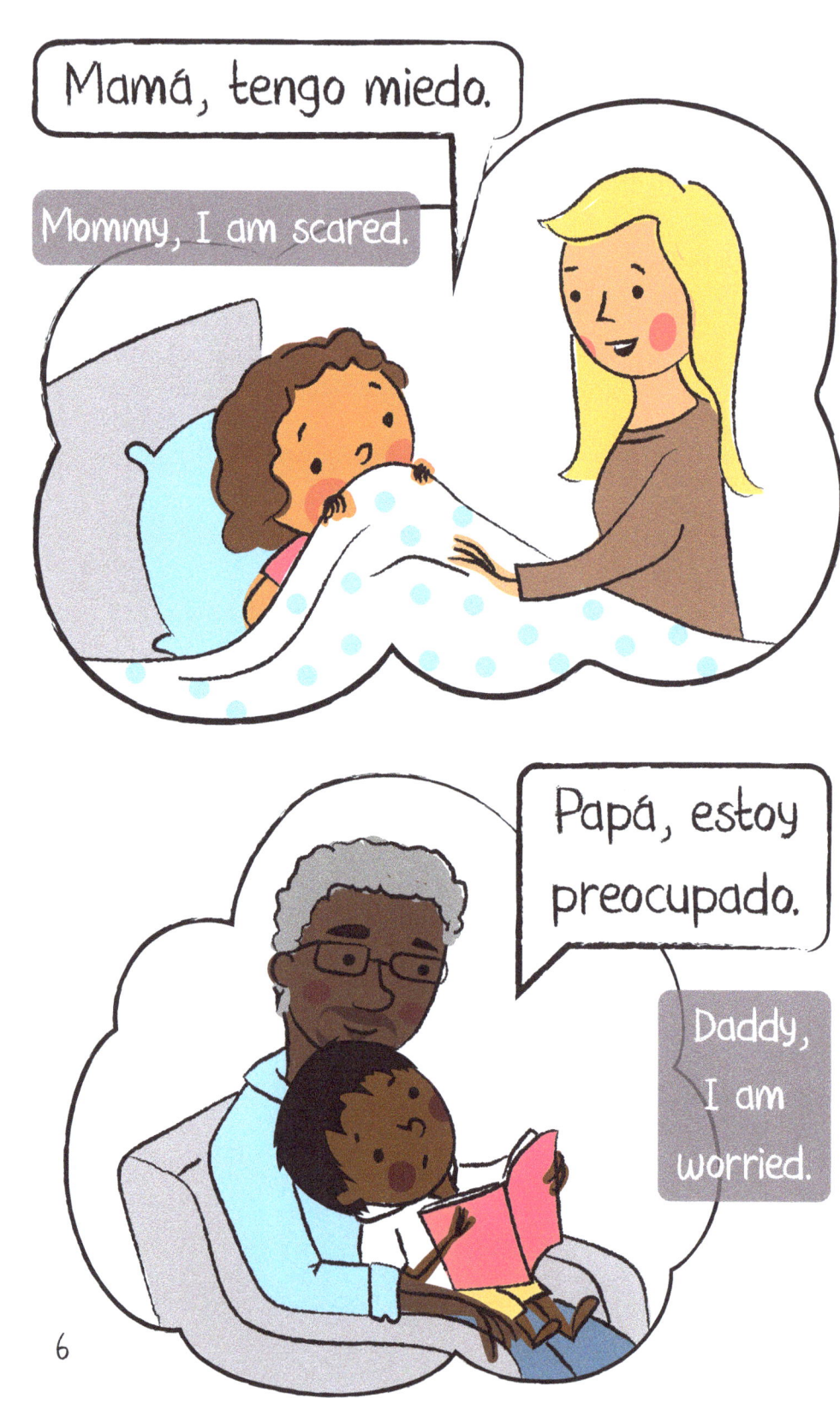

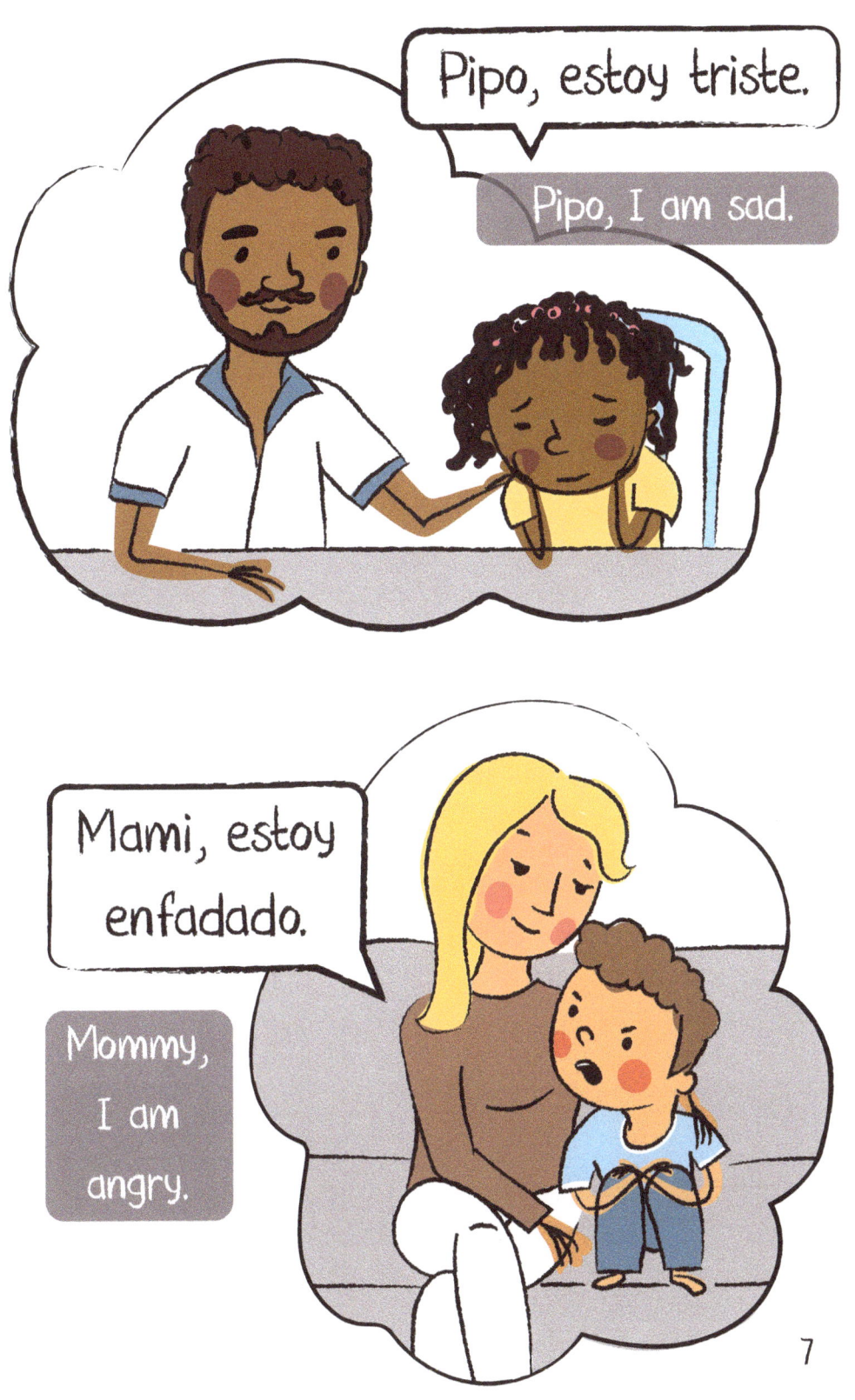

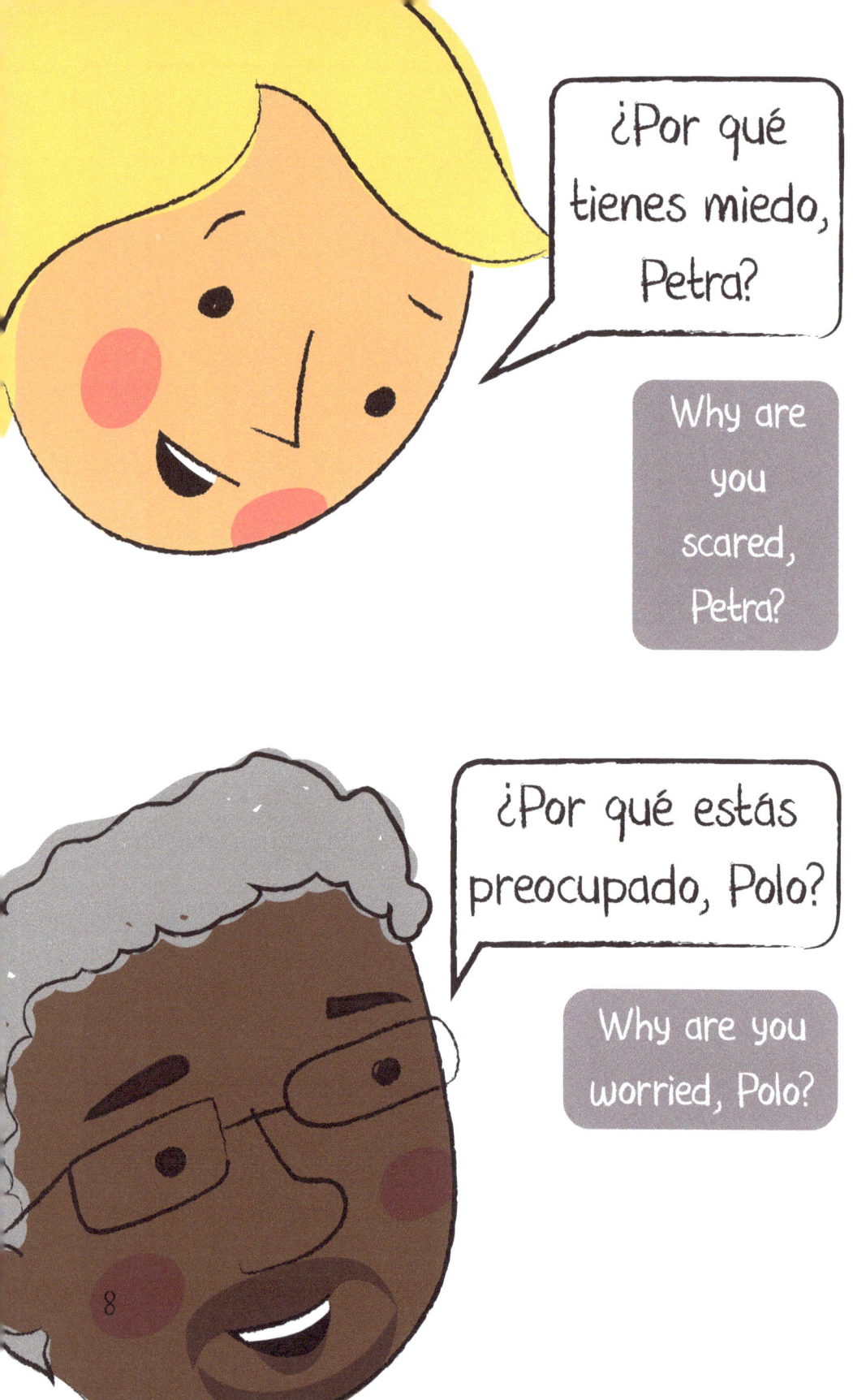

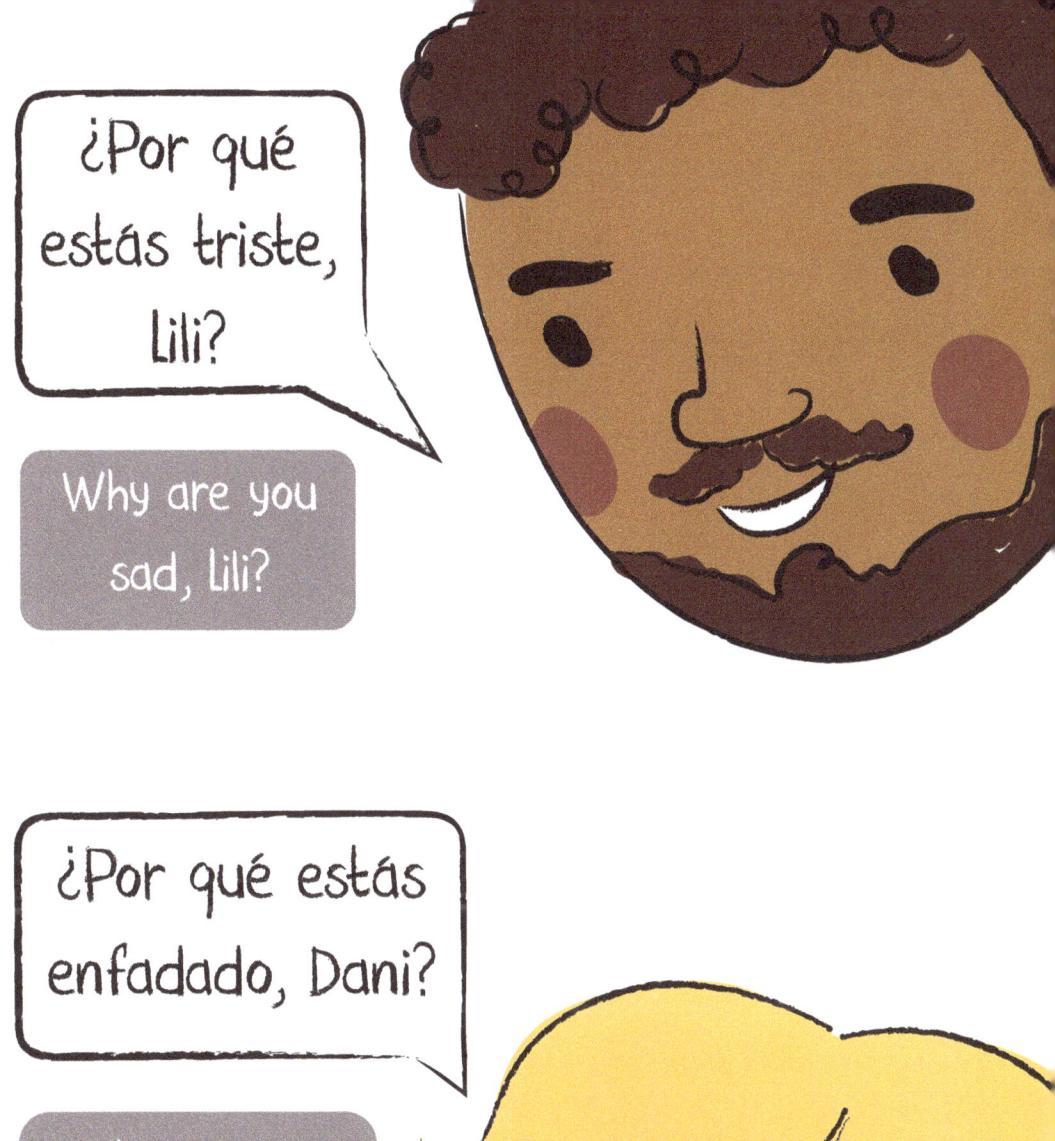

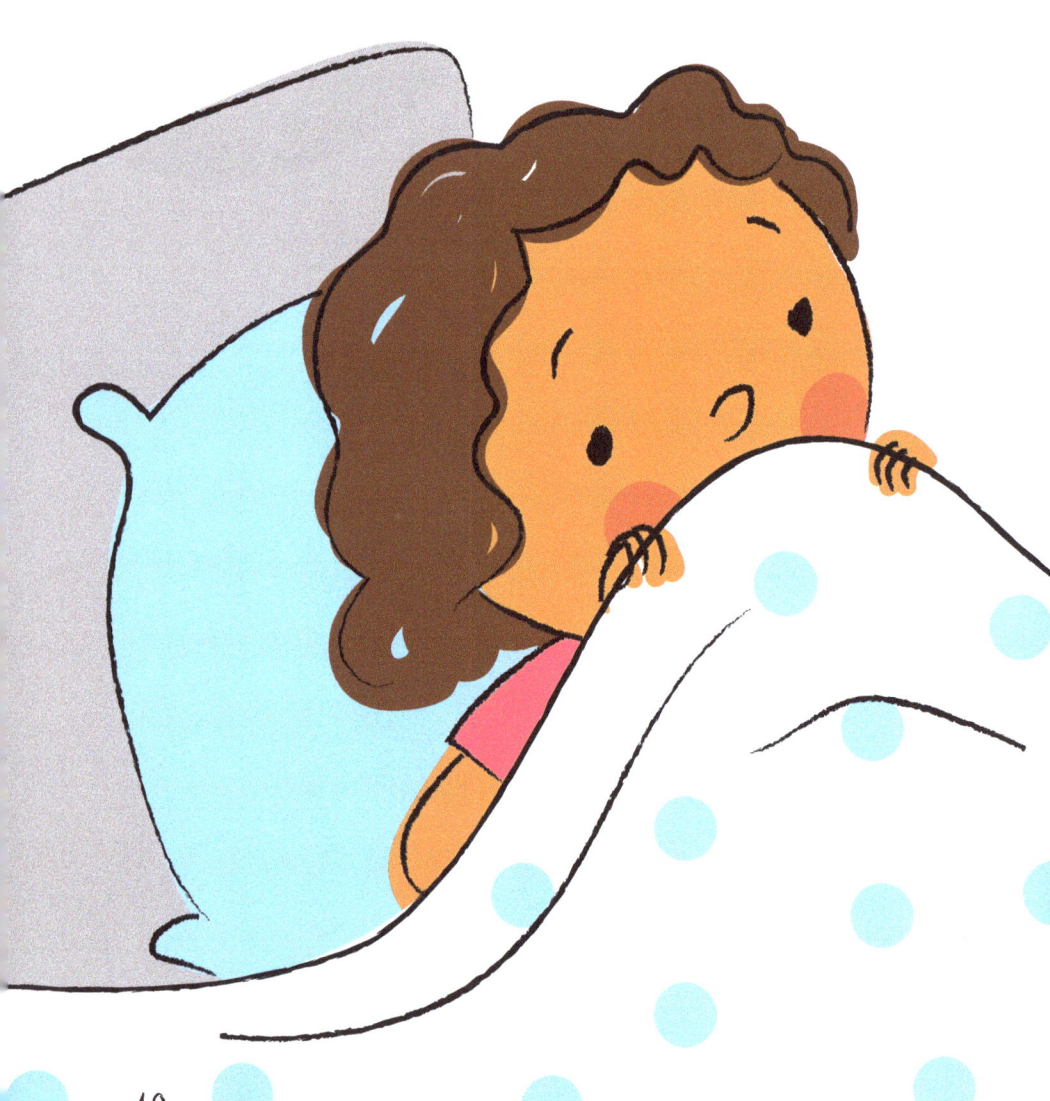

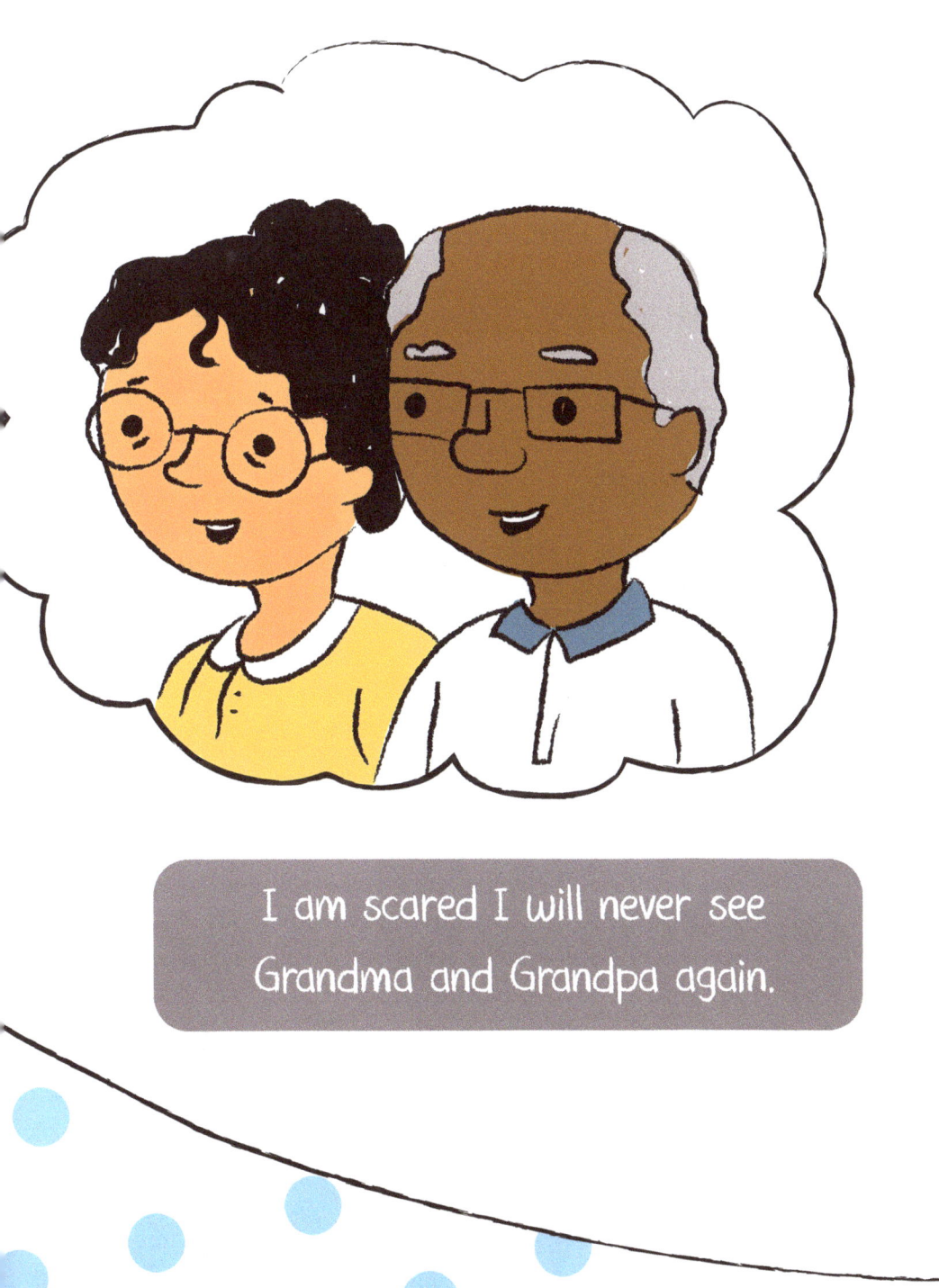

I am scared I will never see Grandma and Grandpa again.

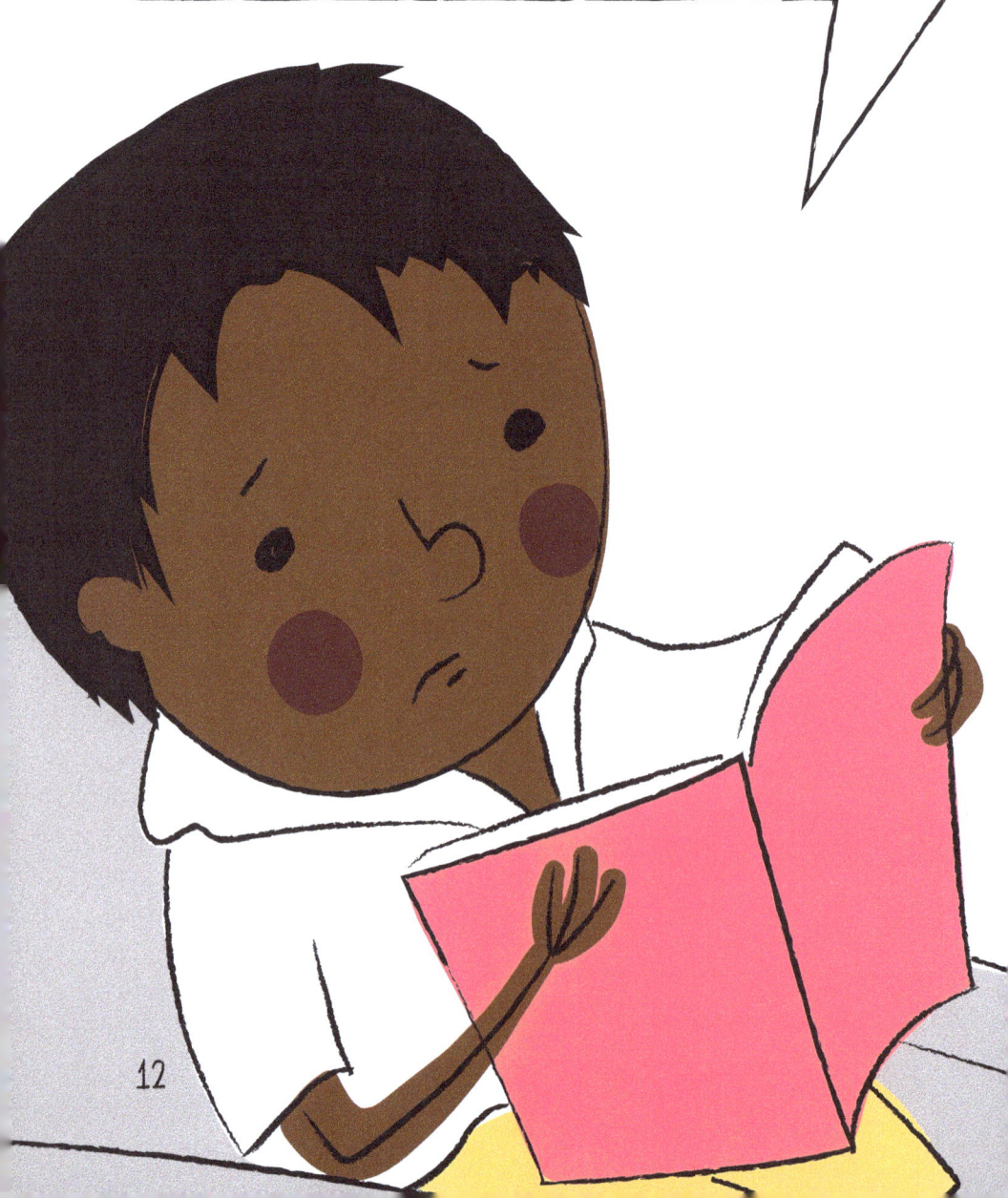

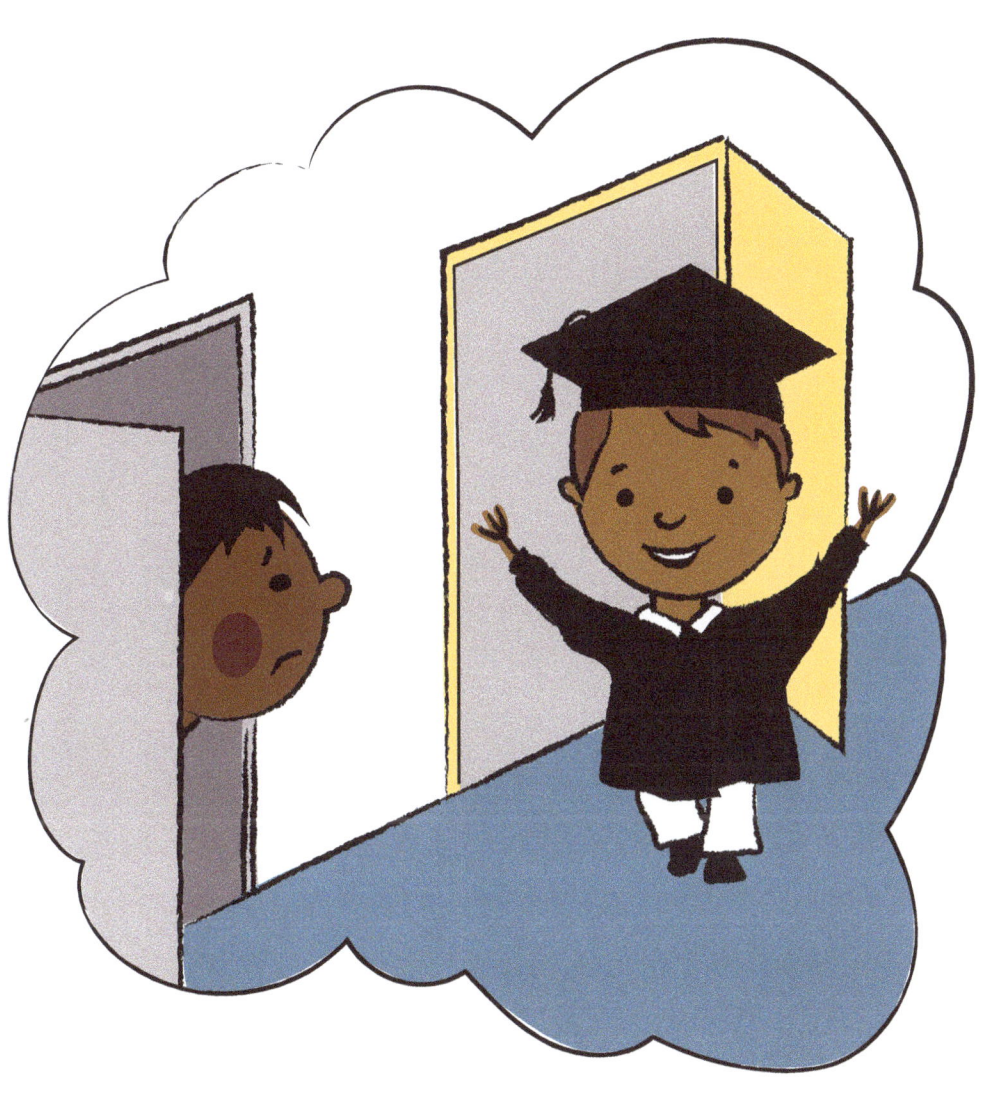

I am worried that I will not be able to graduate because I missed so many days of school.

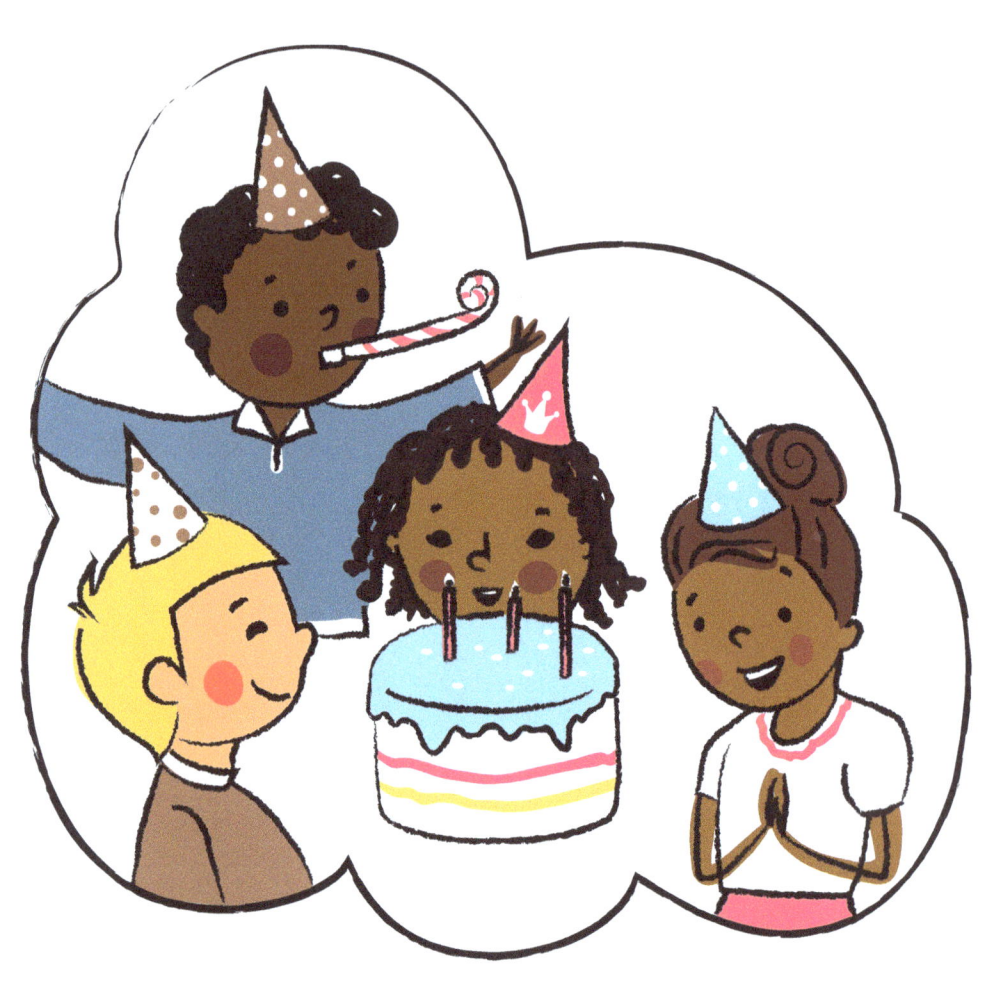

I am sad that I did not get to have a birthday party with my friends this year.

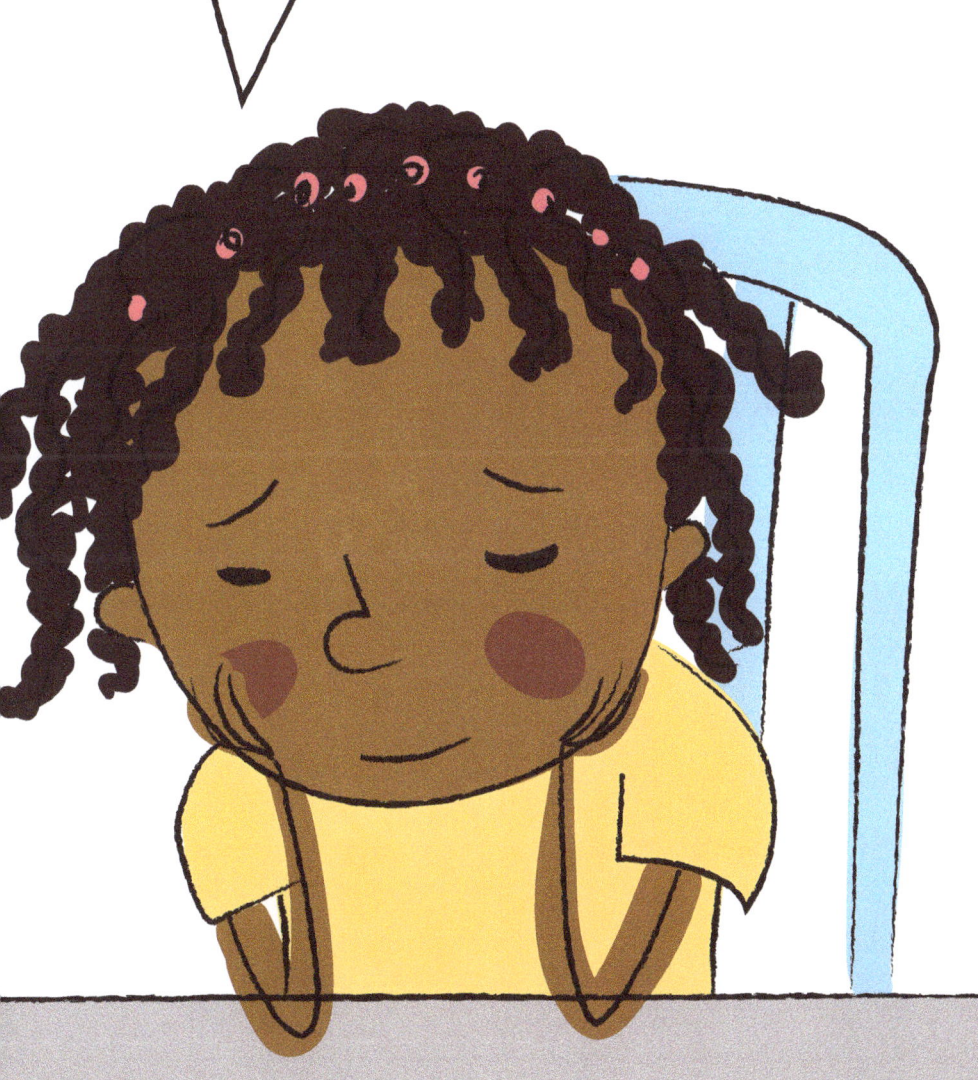

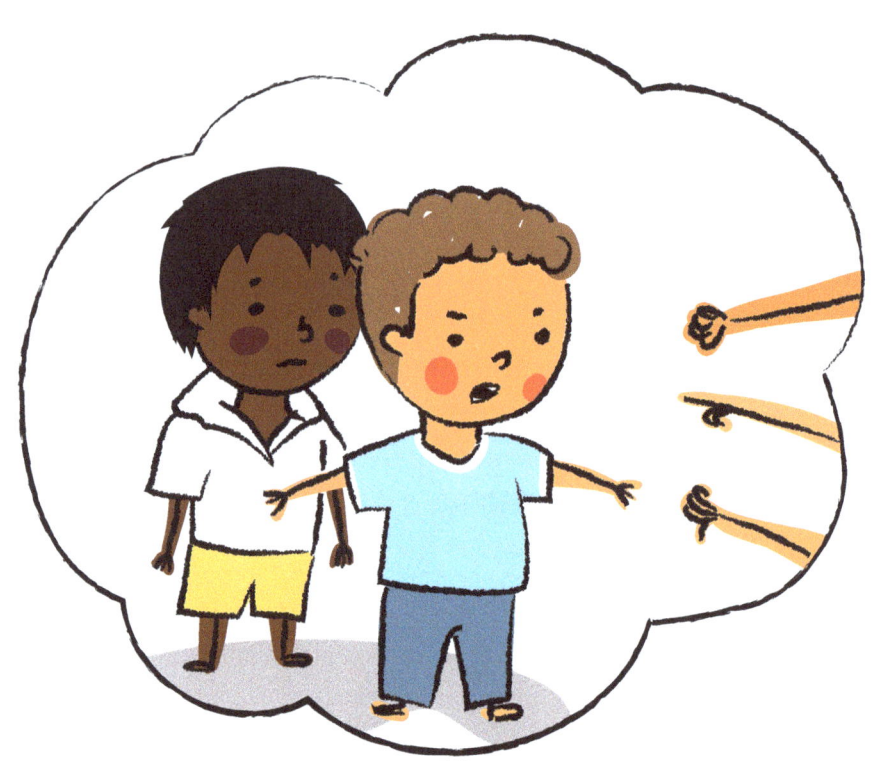

Estoy enfadado porque he visto en la tele que a algunas personas se las trata de manera diferente sólo por el color de su piel. ¡Eso no es justo!

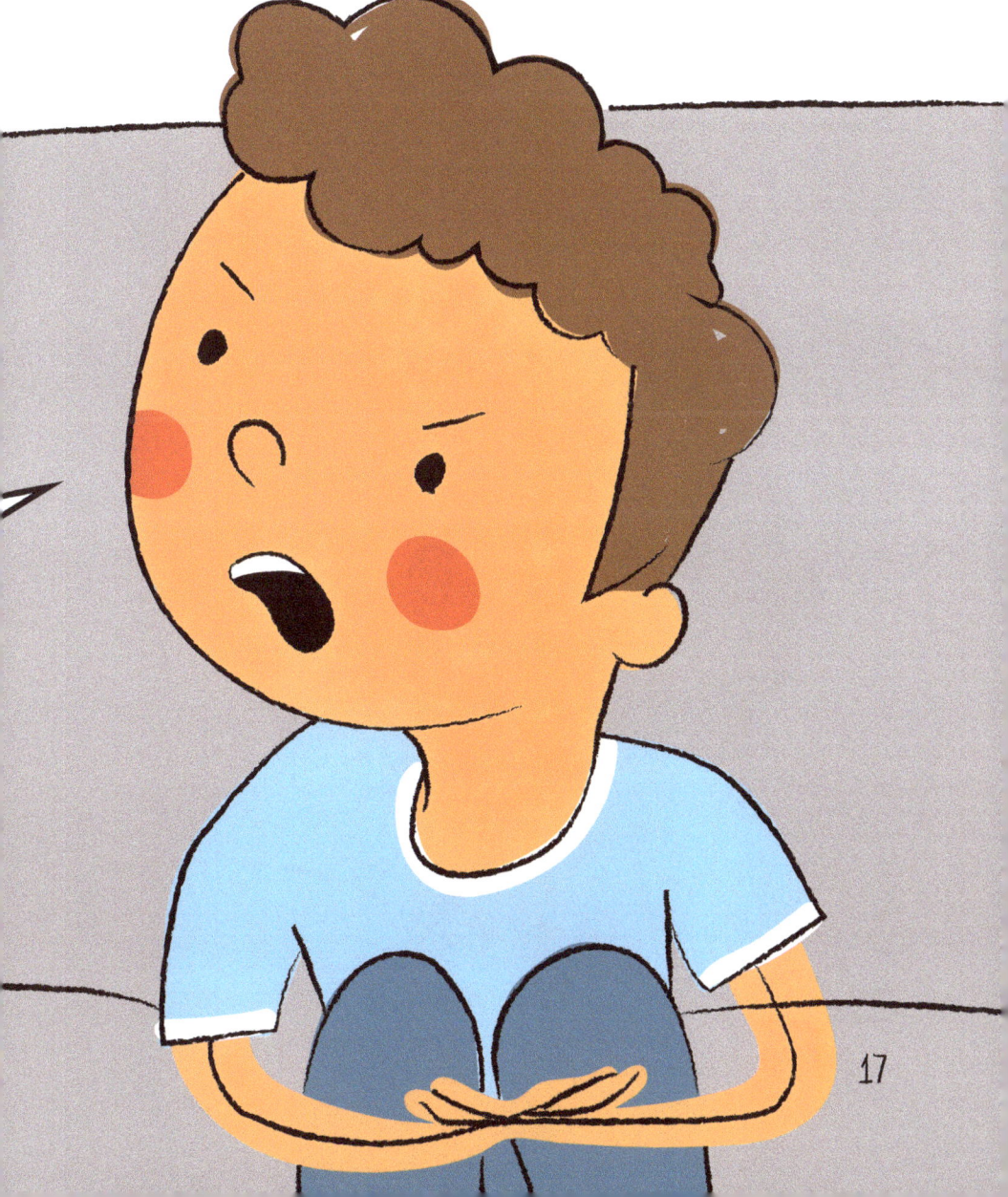

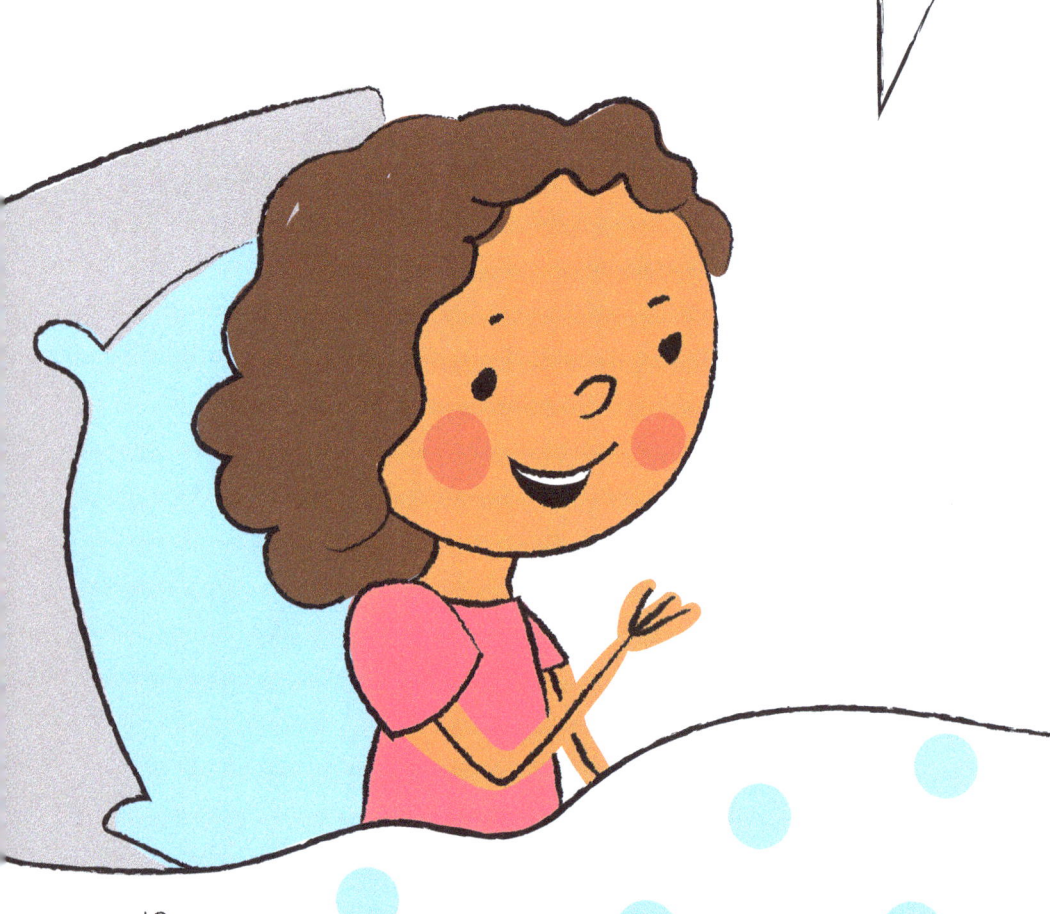

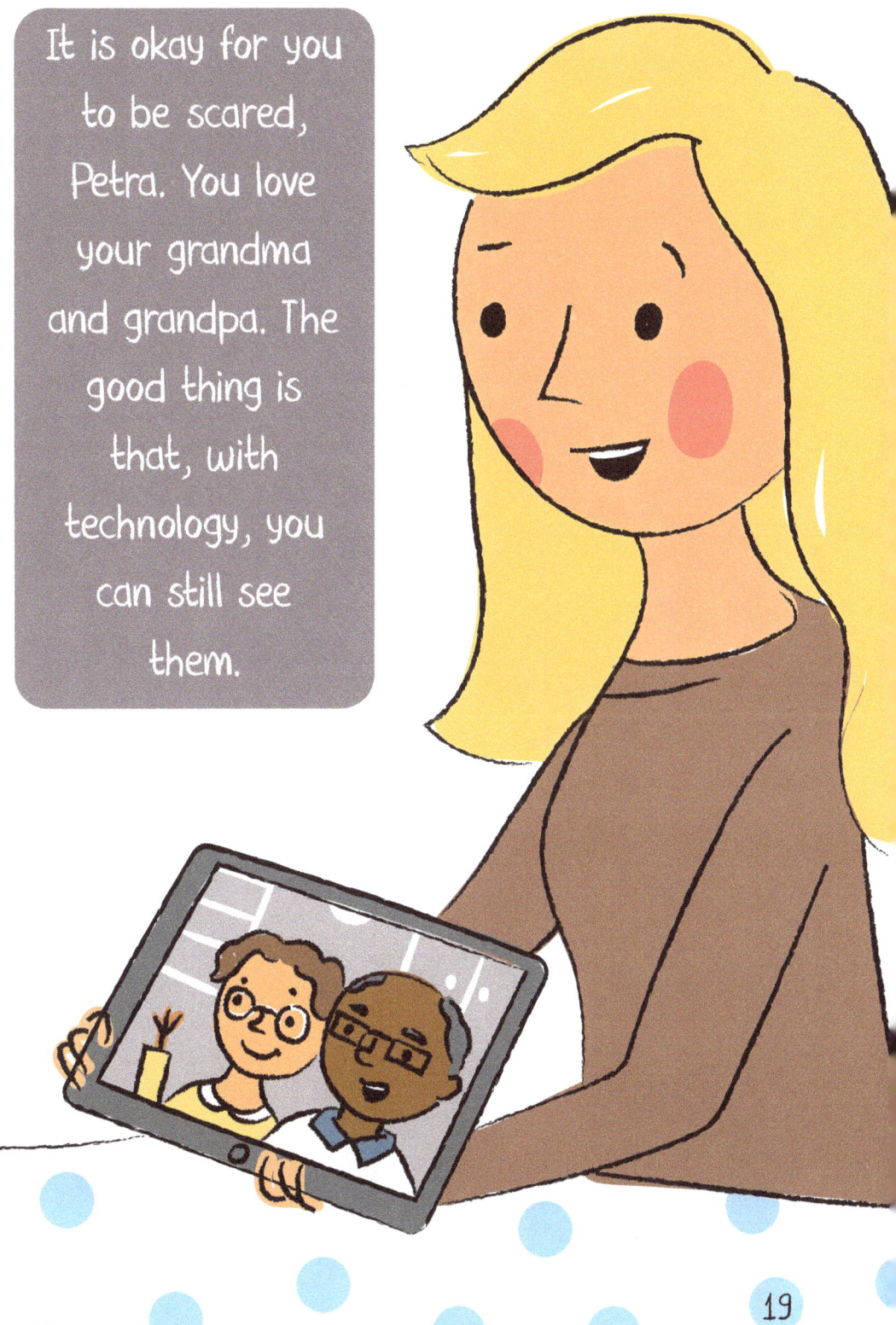

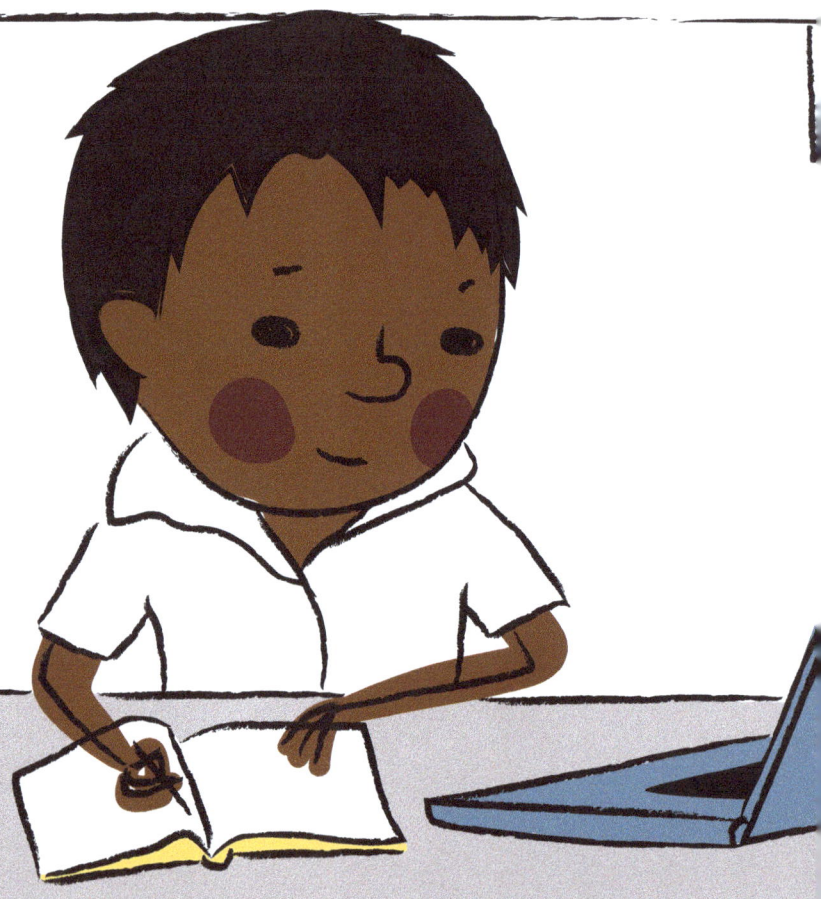

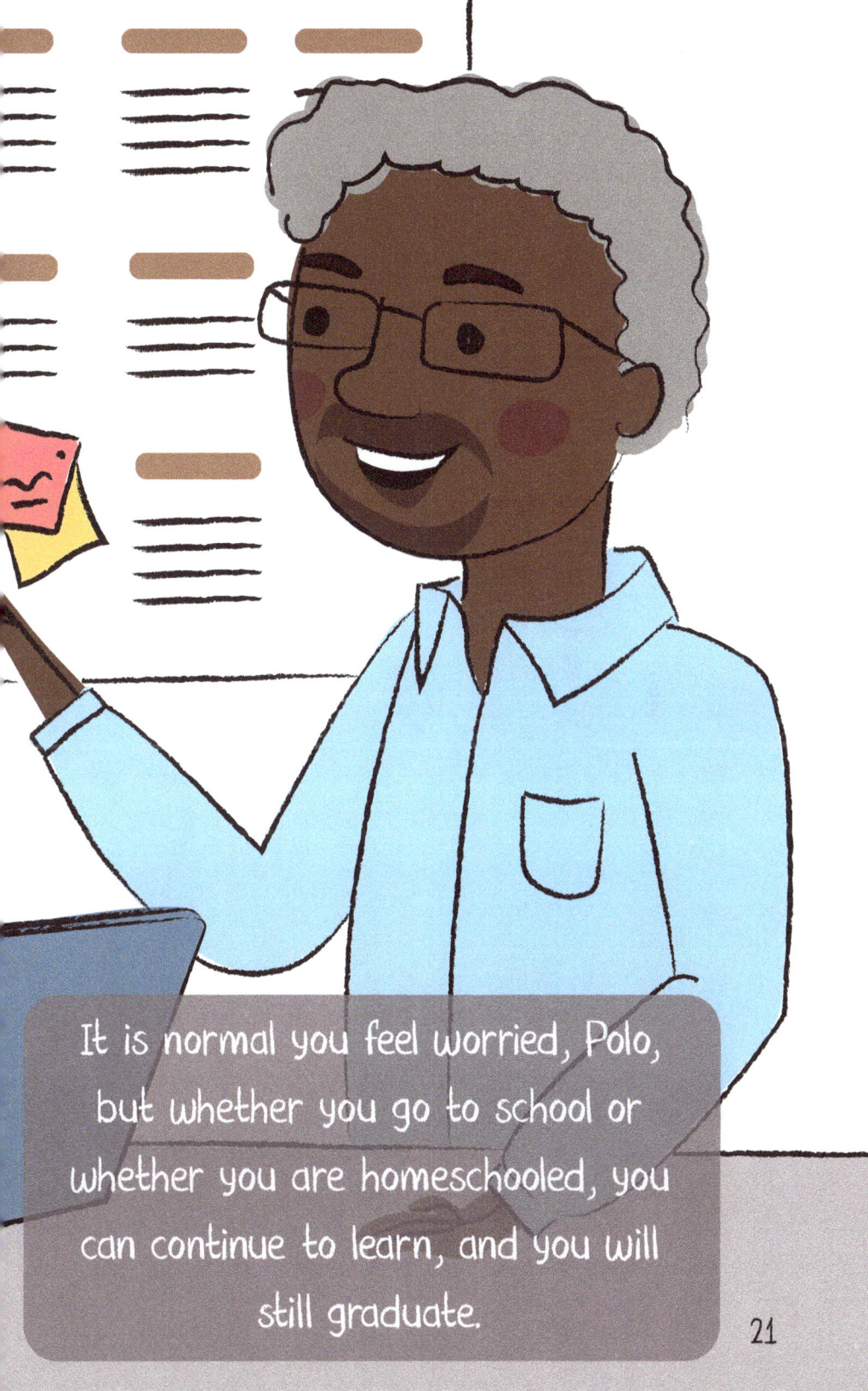

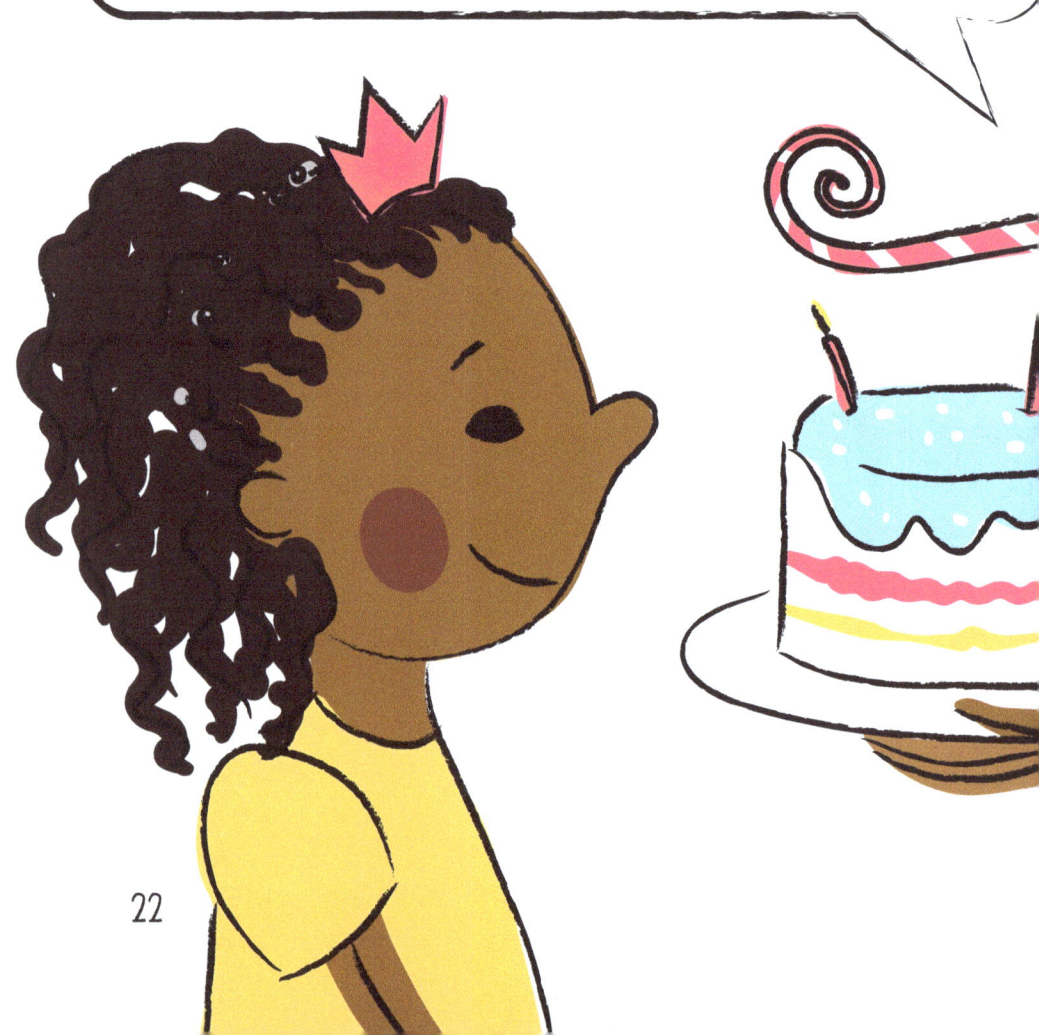

Es normal que estés triste. ¡Llevas mucho tiempo planeando tu fiesta! Este año cortas la tarta con tu familia, que te quiere mucho, pero planearemos una fiesta con tus amigos para el año que viene.

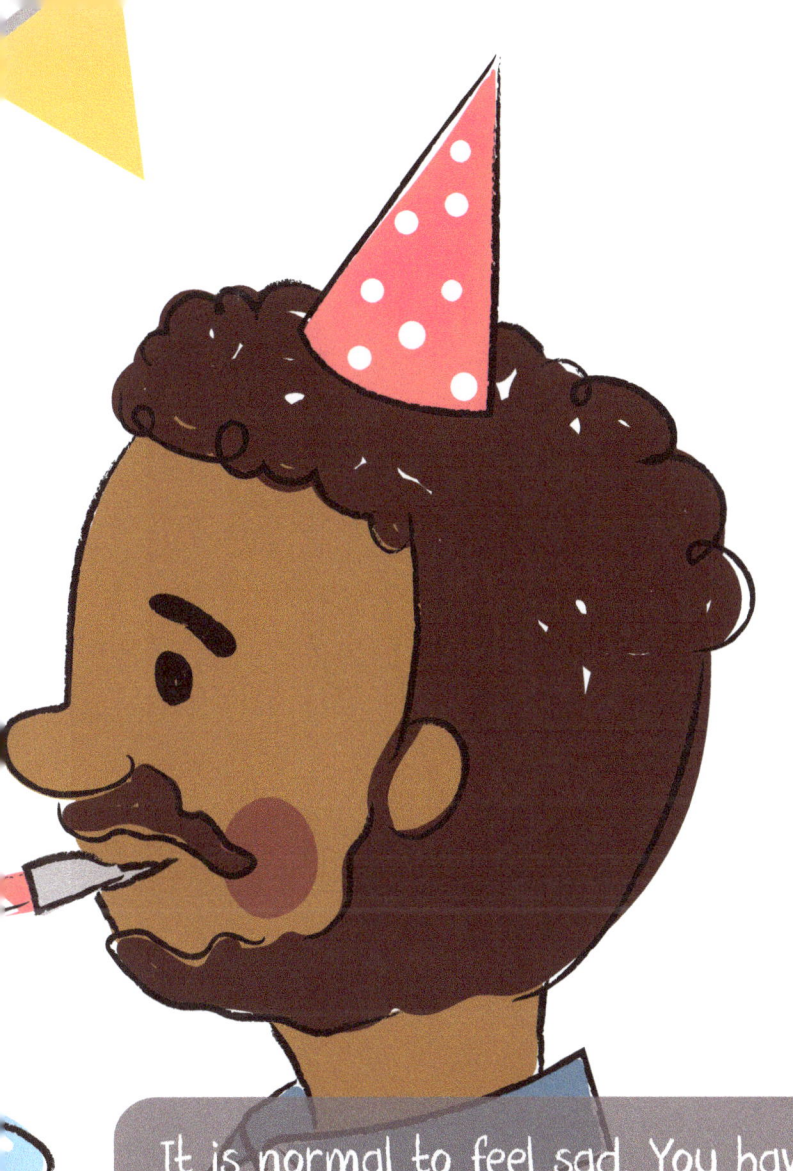

It is normal to feel sad. You have been planning your party for so long! You cut a cake with your family who loves you this year, but we will certainly plan a party with your friends for next year.

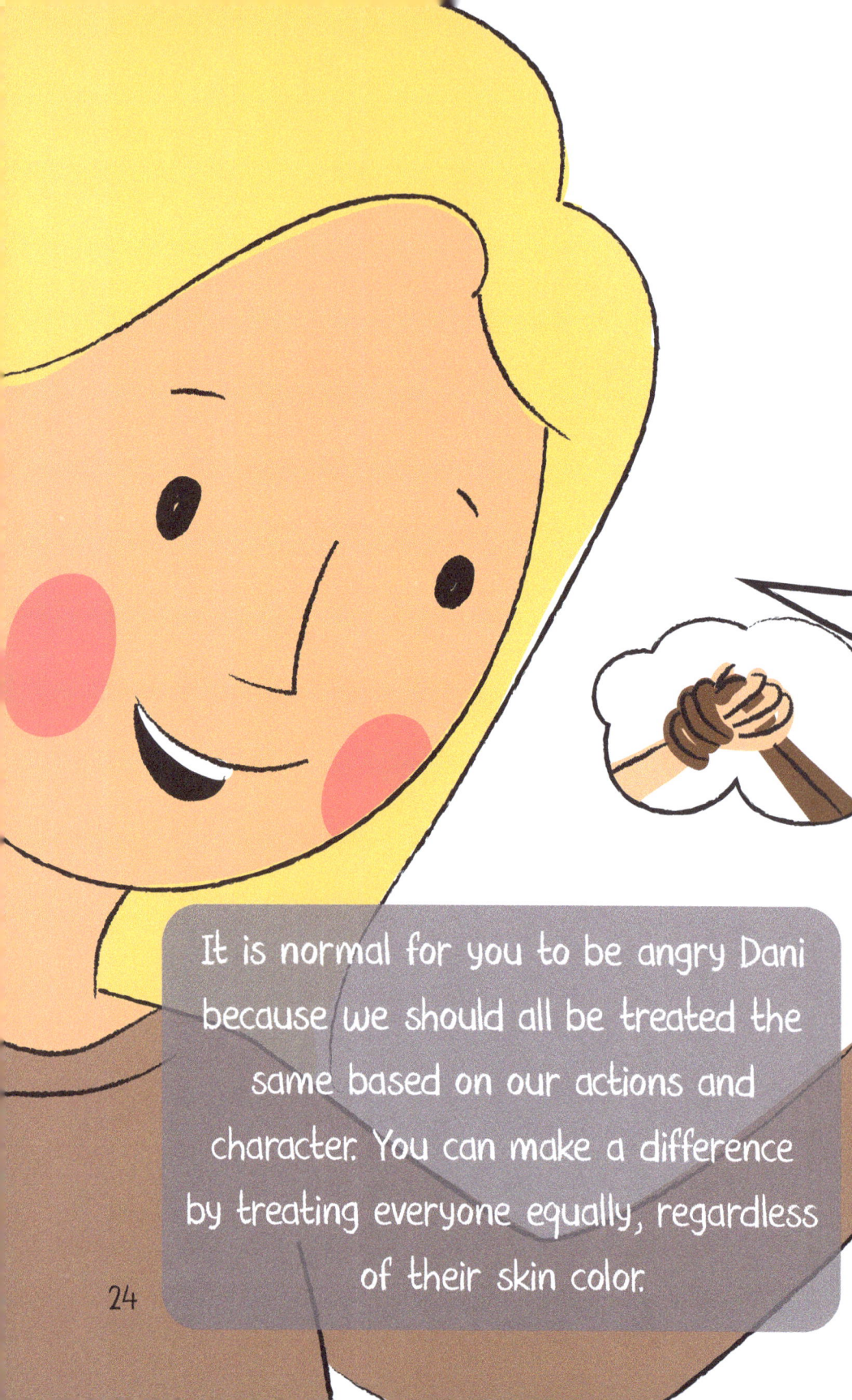

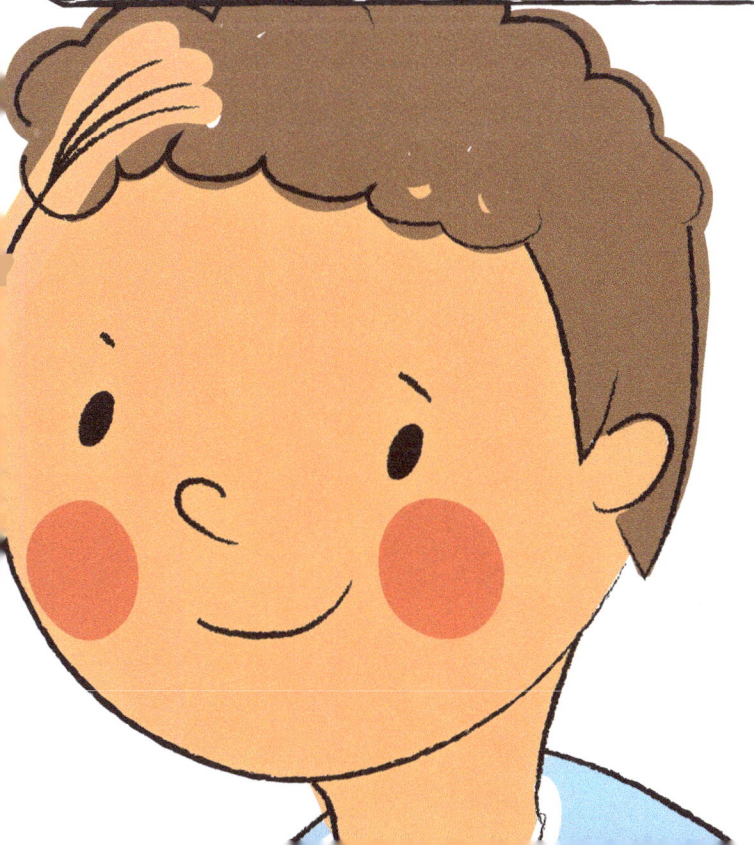

Es normal que estés enfadado, Dani, porque todos deberíamos ser tratados de la misma manera en función de nuestros actos y nuestro carácter. Tú puedes marcar la diferencia tratando a todo el mundo igual, independientemente del color de su piel.

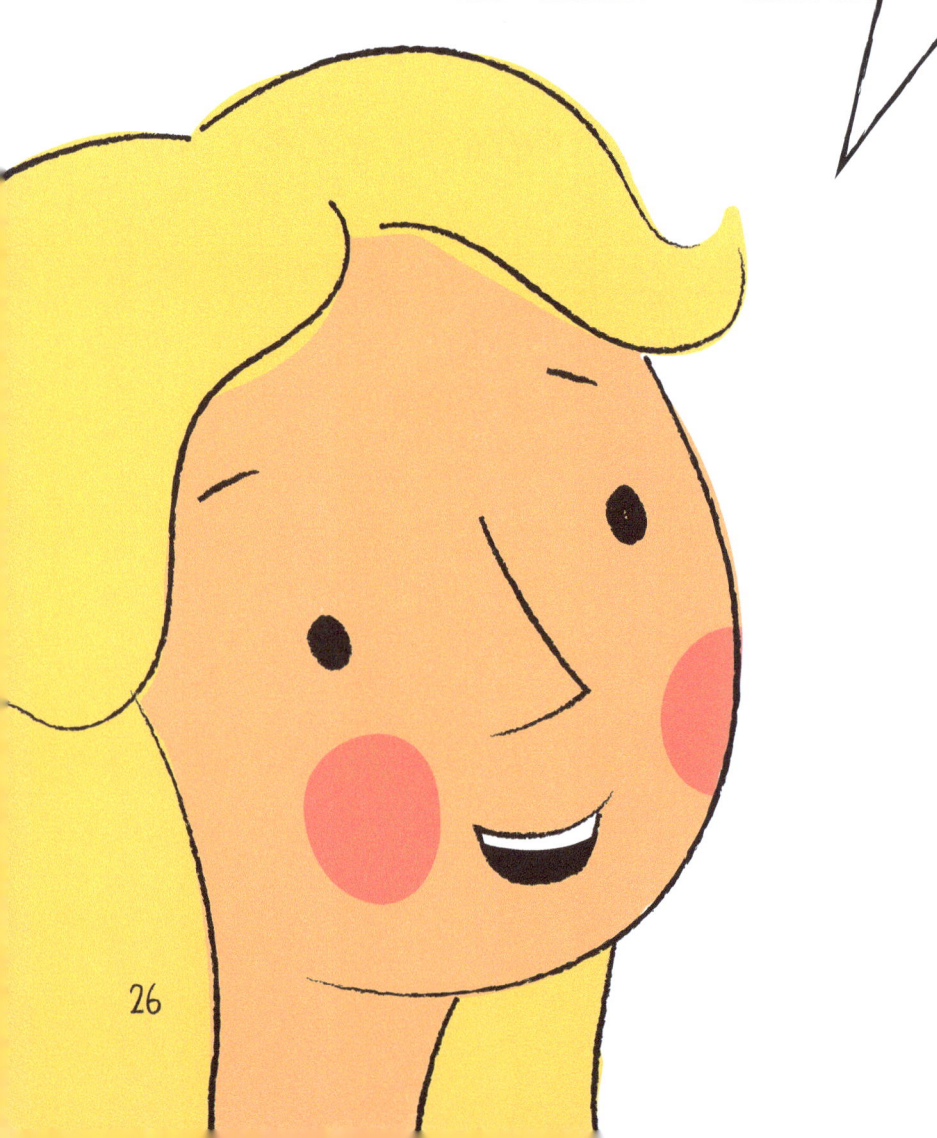

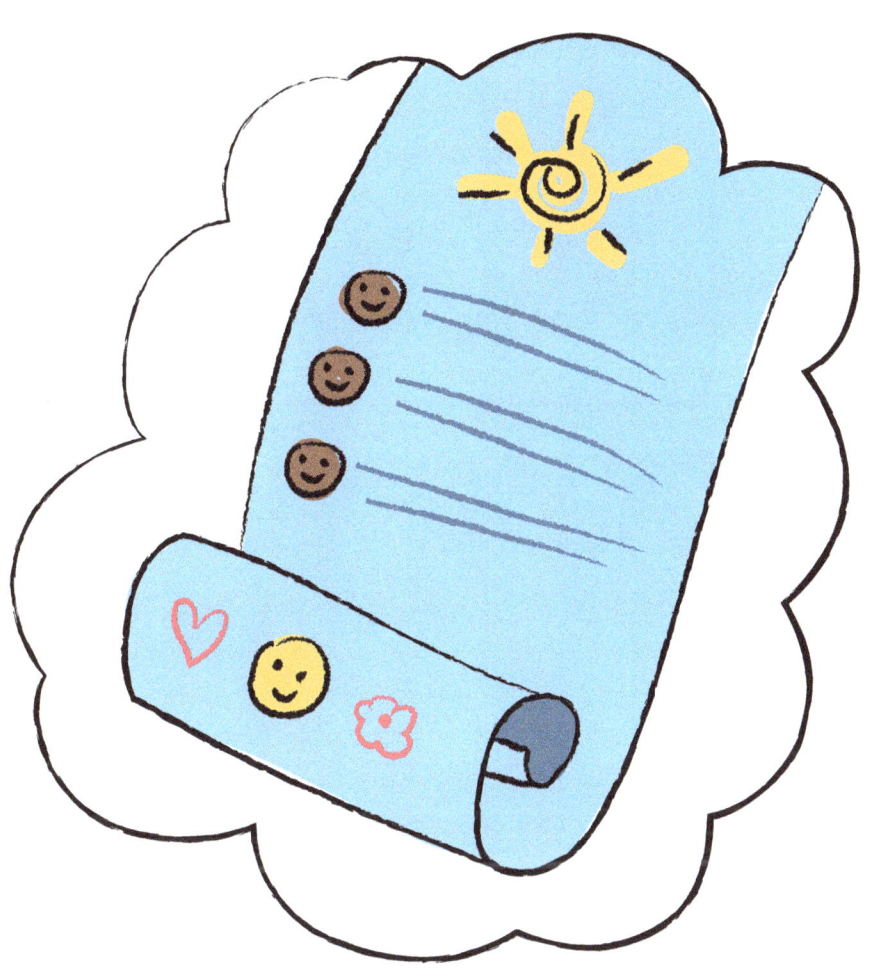

A good way to feel better when you are scared, sad, worried or angry is to make a list of everything you are grateful for.

¿Qué significa estar agradecido?

What does it mean to be grateful?

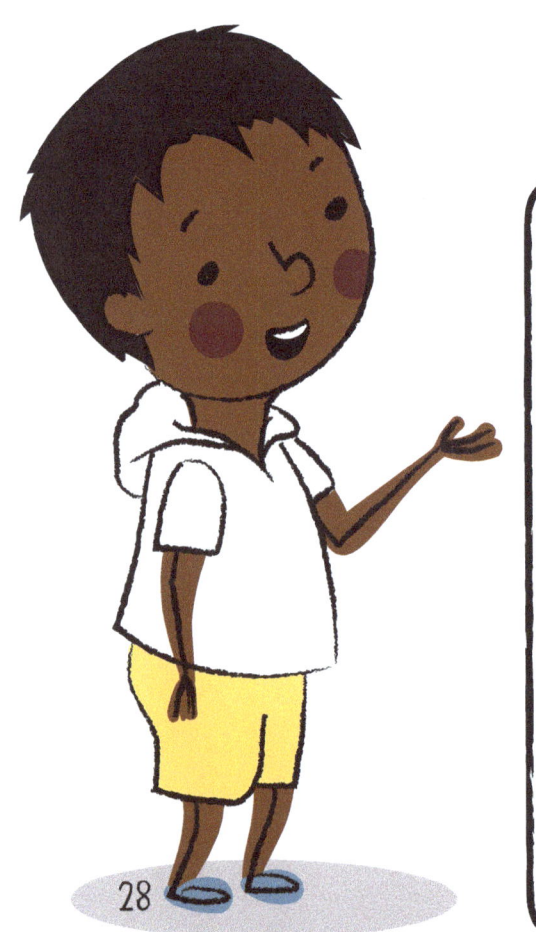

Significa expresar gratitud. En otras palabras, decir "gracias" por las cosas que tienes en tu vida.

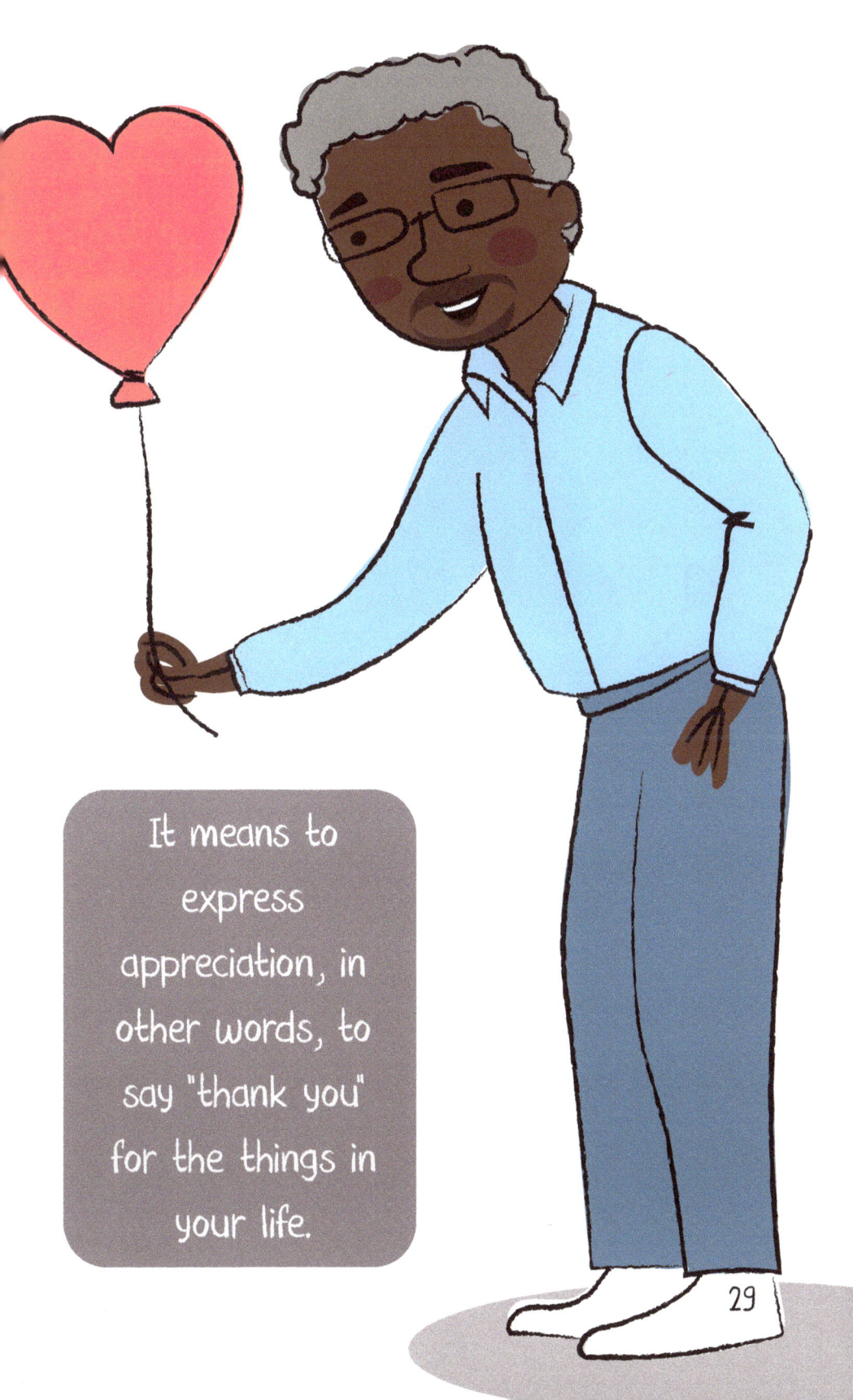

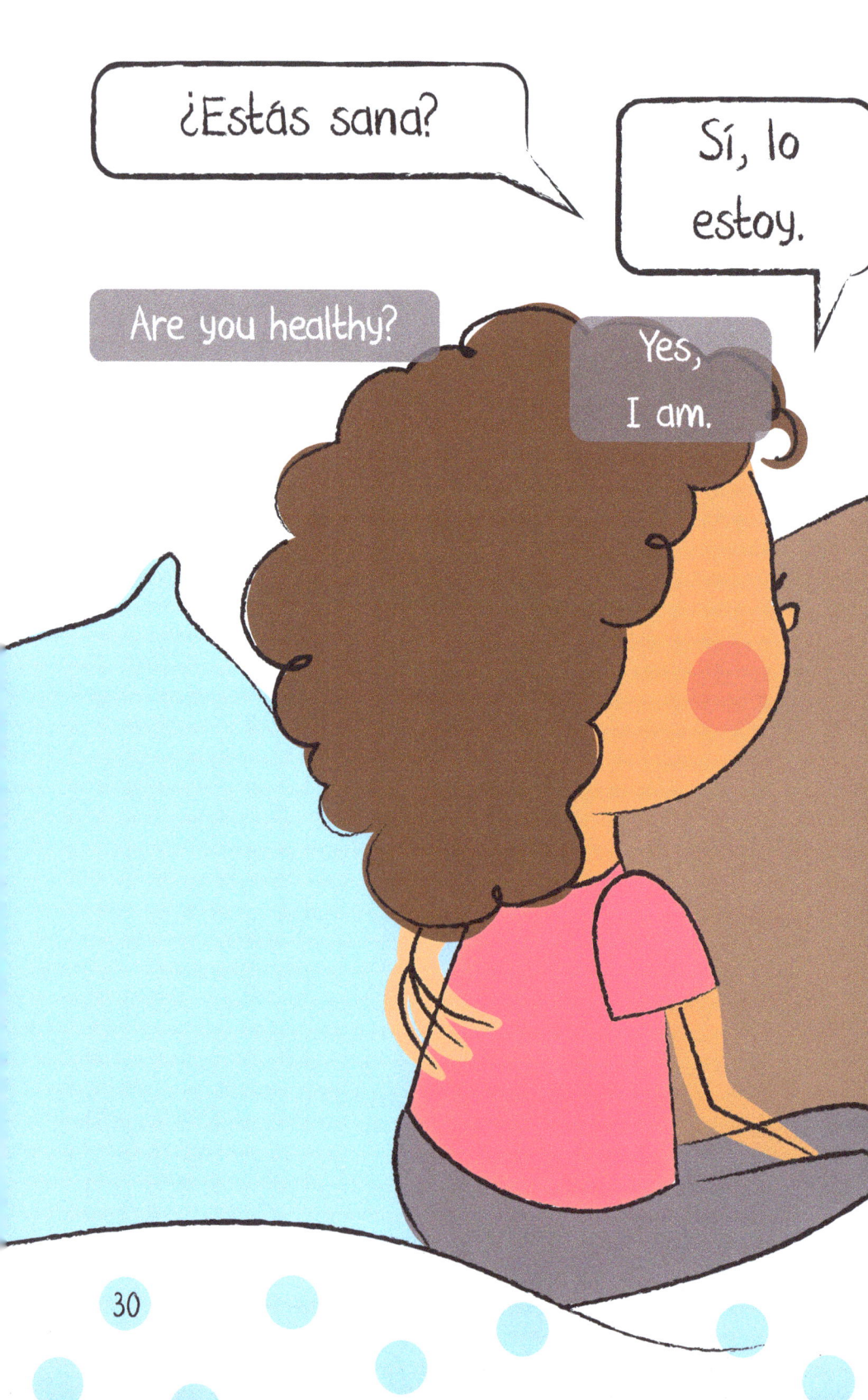

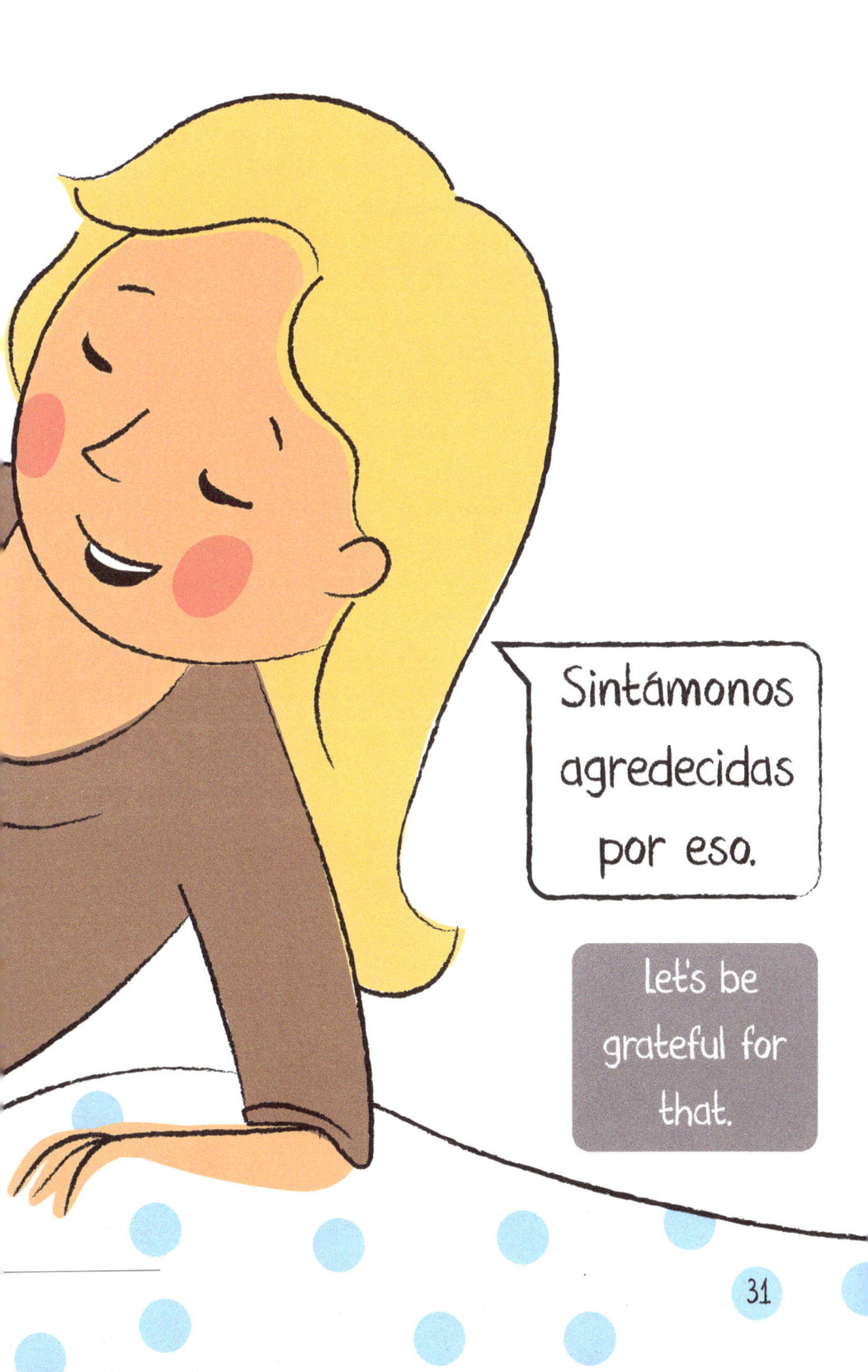

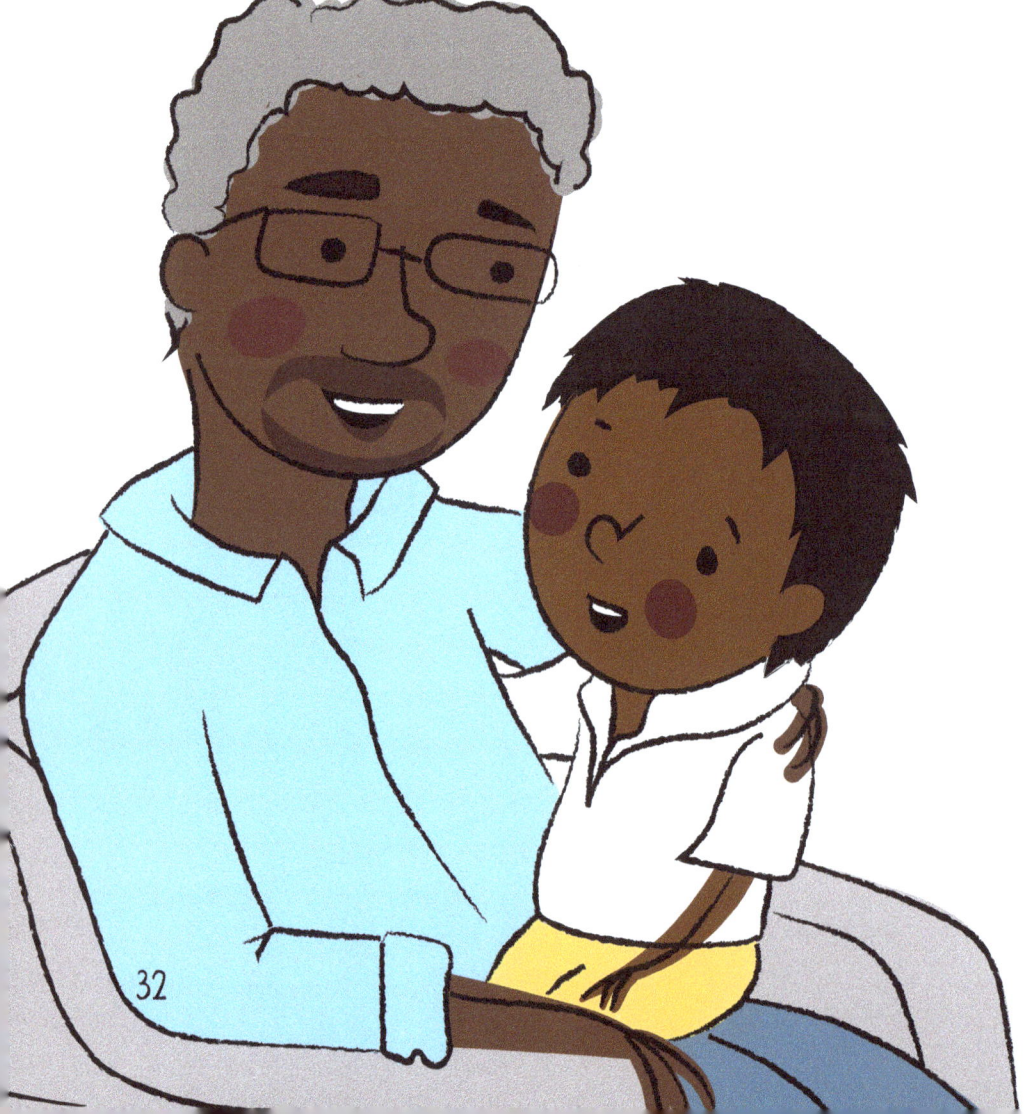

Sí, ¡mi profesor nos envió un video genial sobre los planetas del sistema solar!

Yes, my teacher assigned to us a cool video about the solar planets!

¡Guau! ¿No es eso algo por lo que sentirse agradecido?

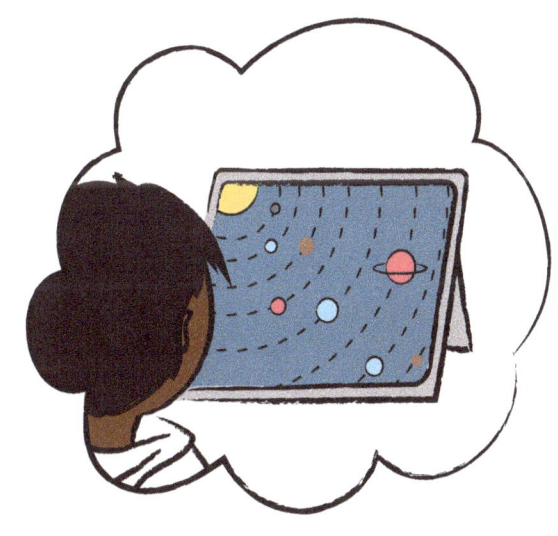

Wow! Isn't that something to be grateful for?!

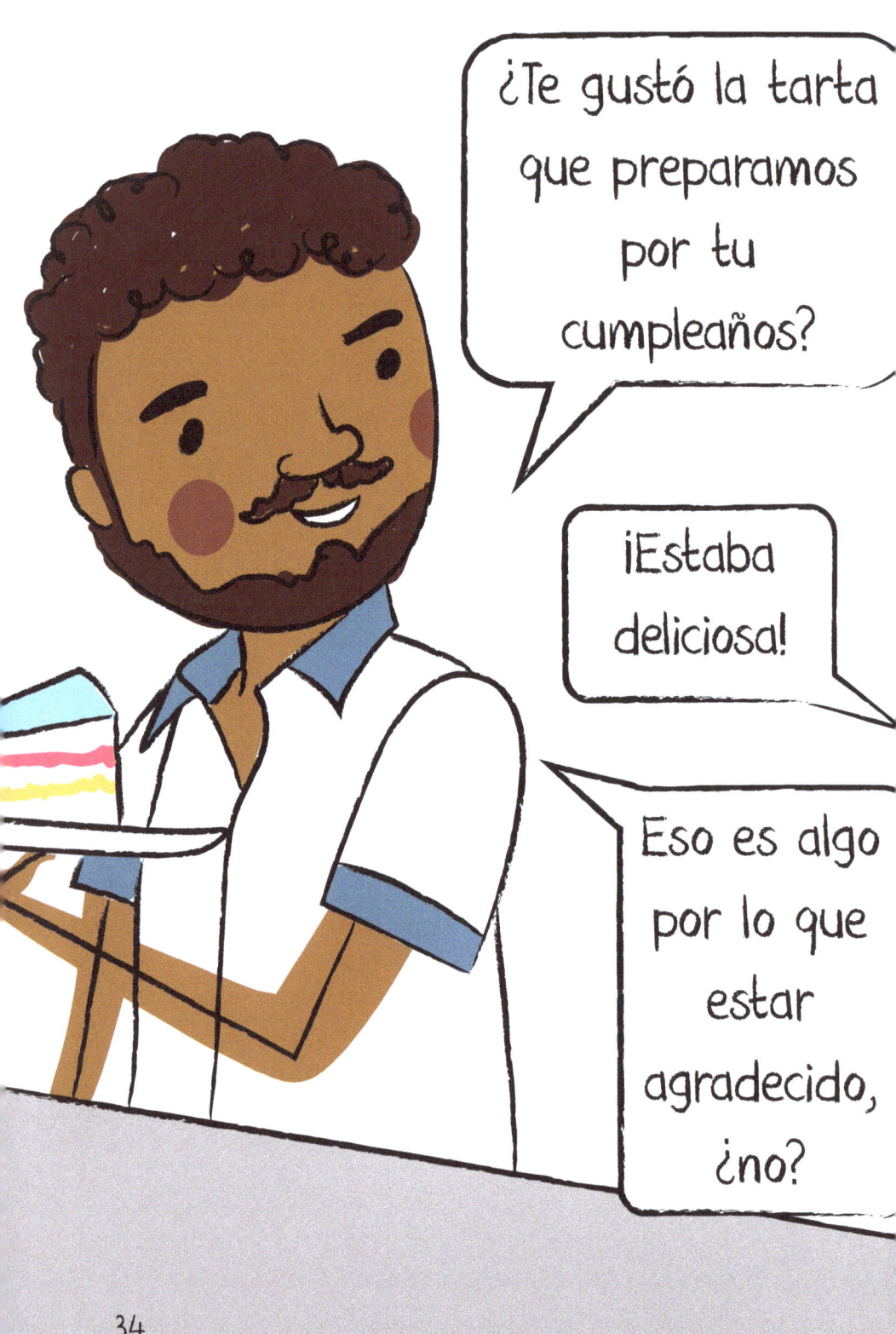

How did you like the cake we baked for your birthday?

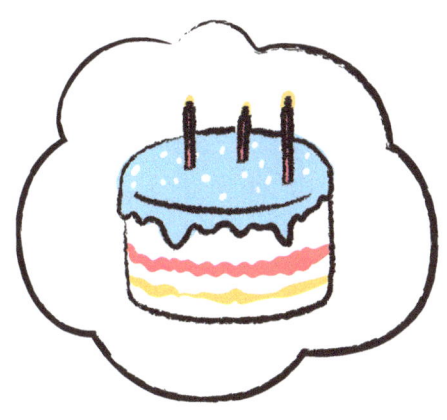

It was delicious!

That is something to be grateful for, don't you think?

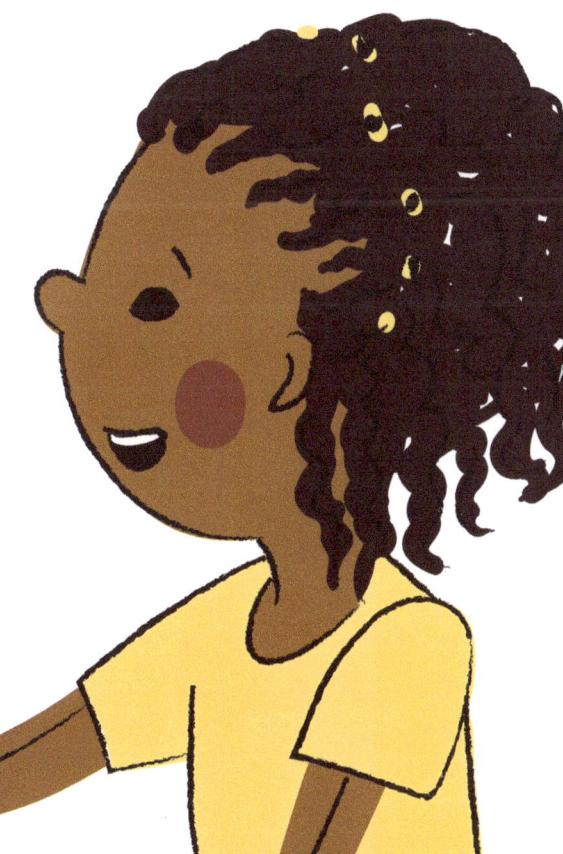

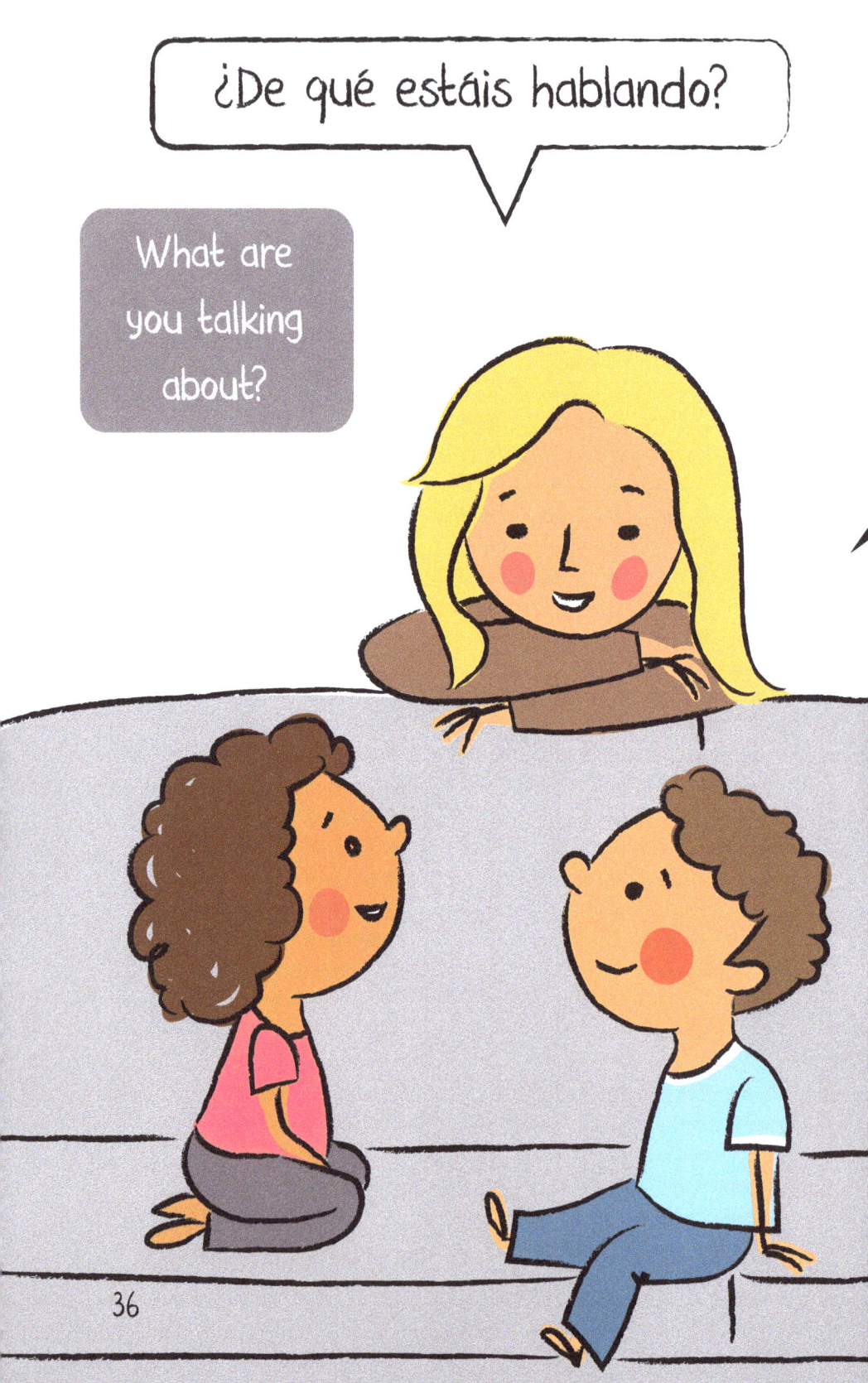

Hemos visto en la tele a gente de todo el mundo marchando para garantizar que todas las personas sean tratadas igual.

We saw on TV people around the world marching to ensure that everyone is treated equally regardless of their skin color.

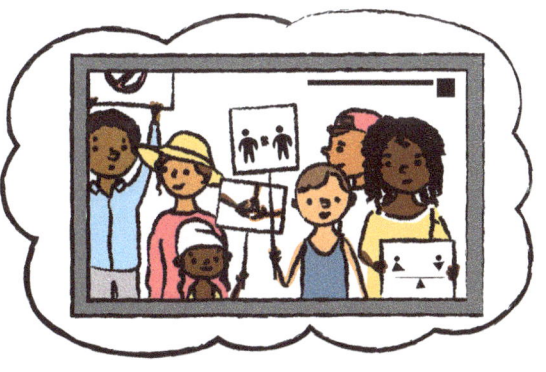

Eso es un motivo para estar muy agradecido.

That is so much to be grateful for.

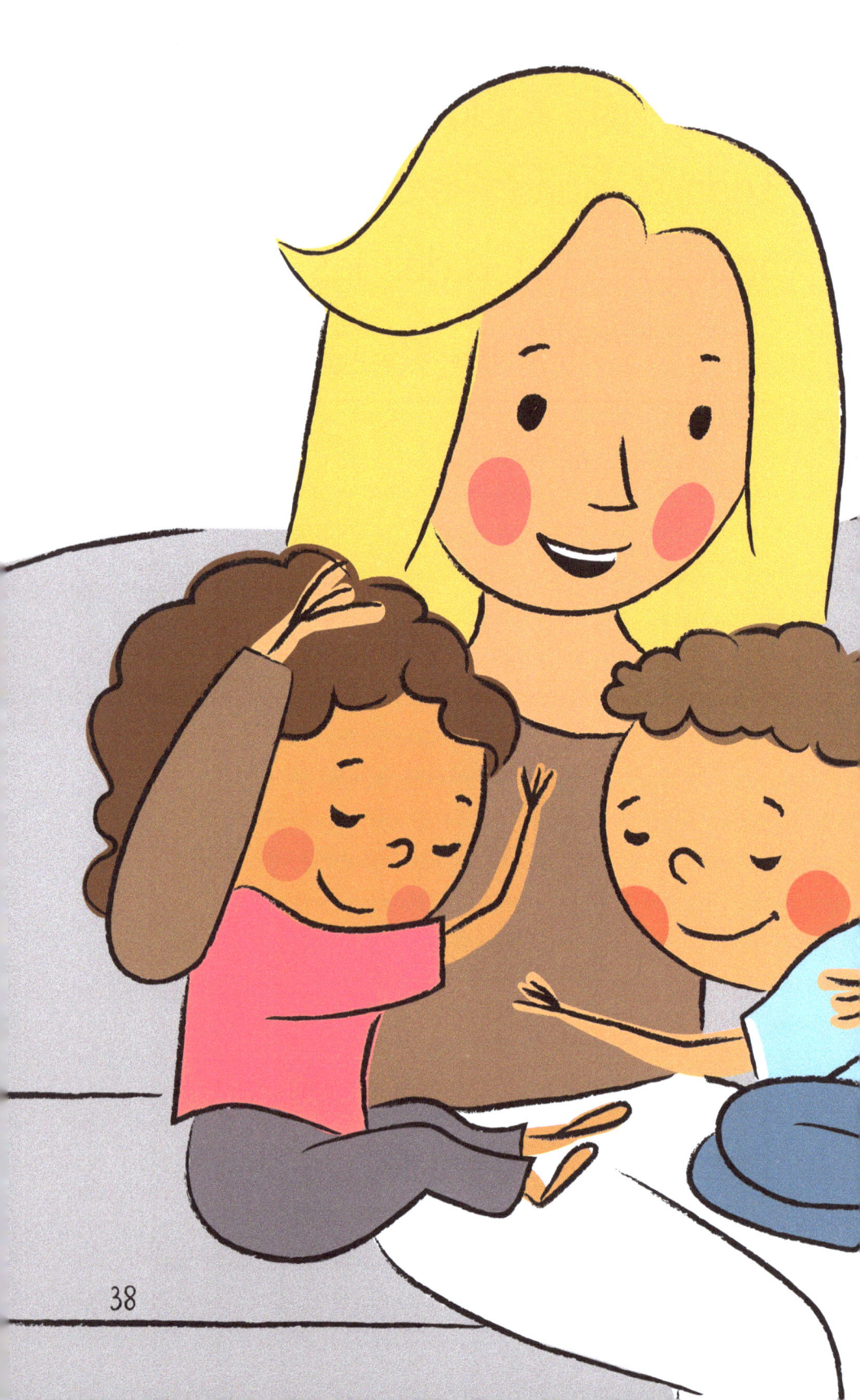

Cuando hay cambios e inseguridad, es normal sentirse asustado, triste, preocupado o, incluso, enfadado. Sin embargo, ayuda hablar sobre ello.

When there is uncertainty and change, it is normal to feel scared, sad, worried or even angry. However, it helps to talk about it.

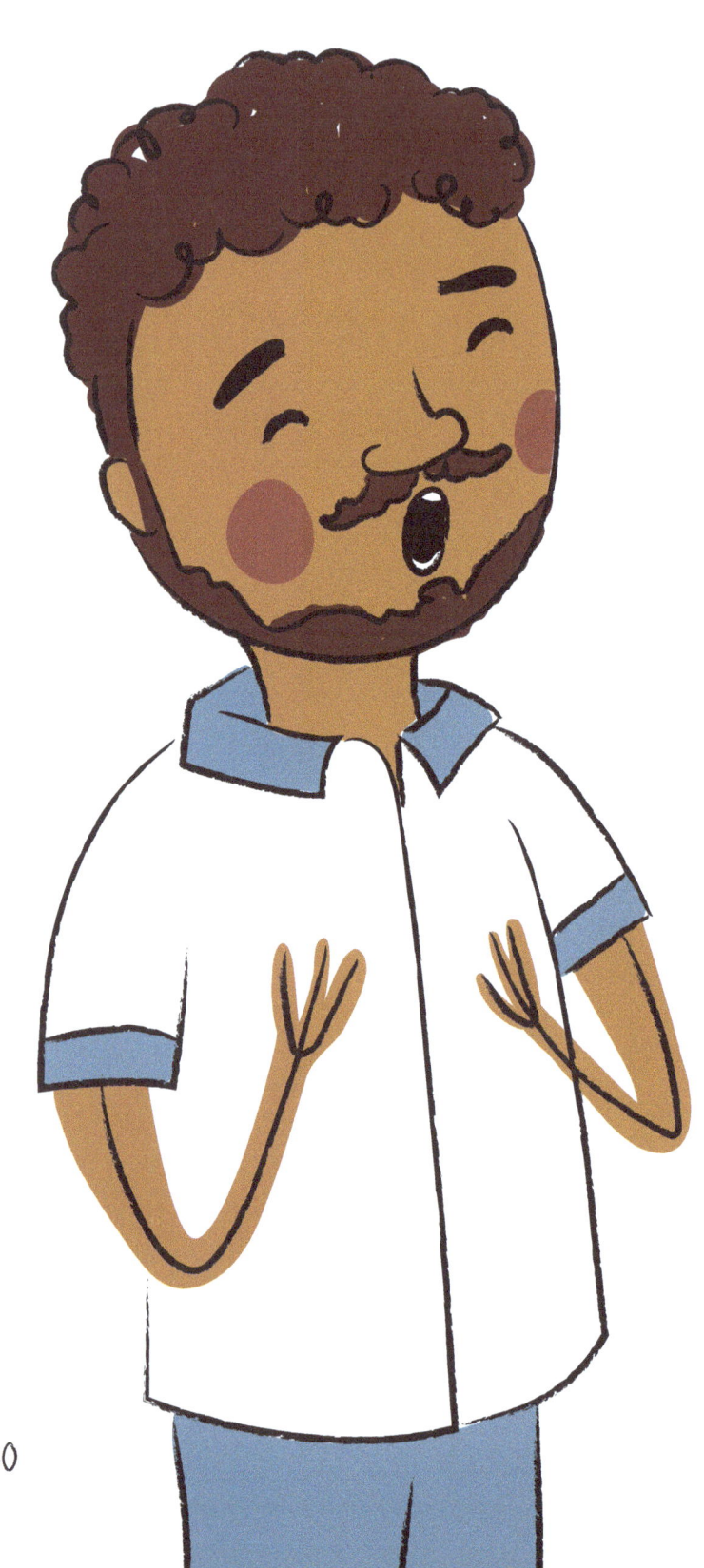

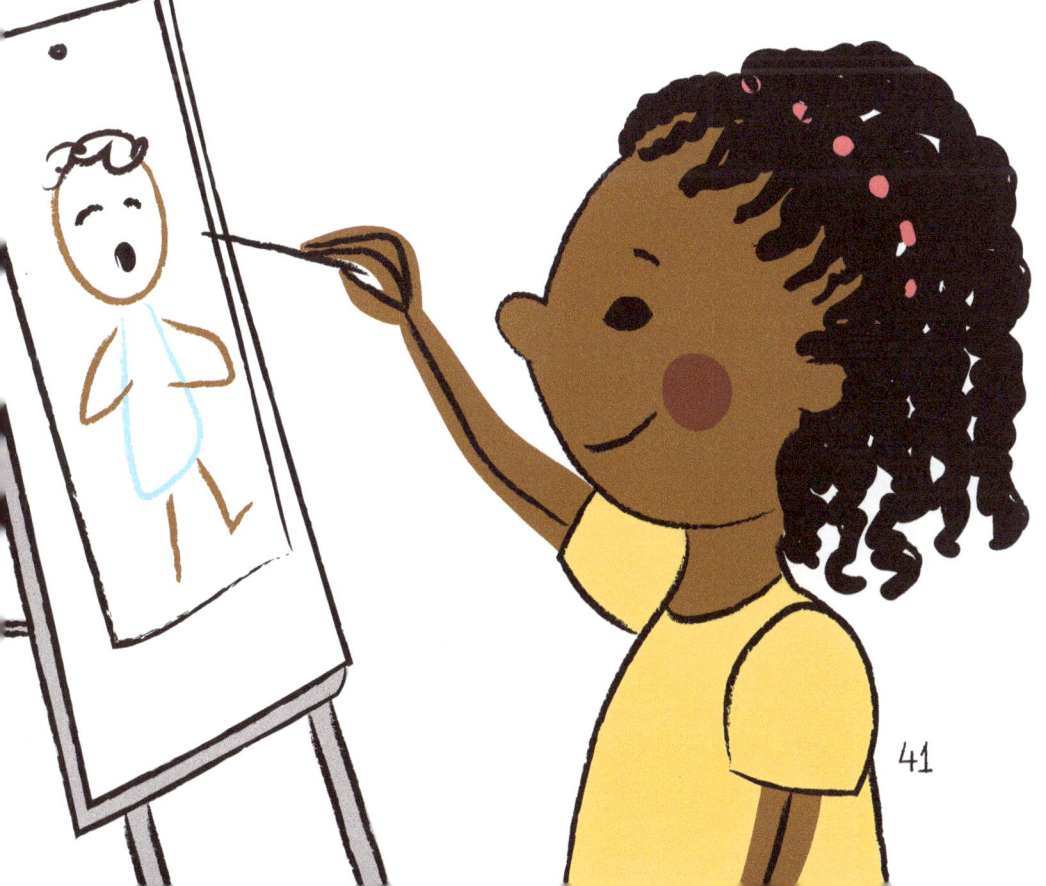

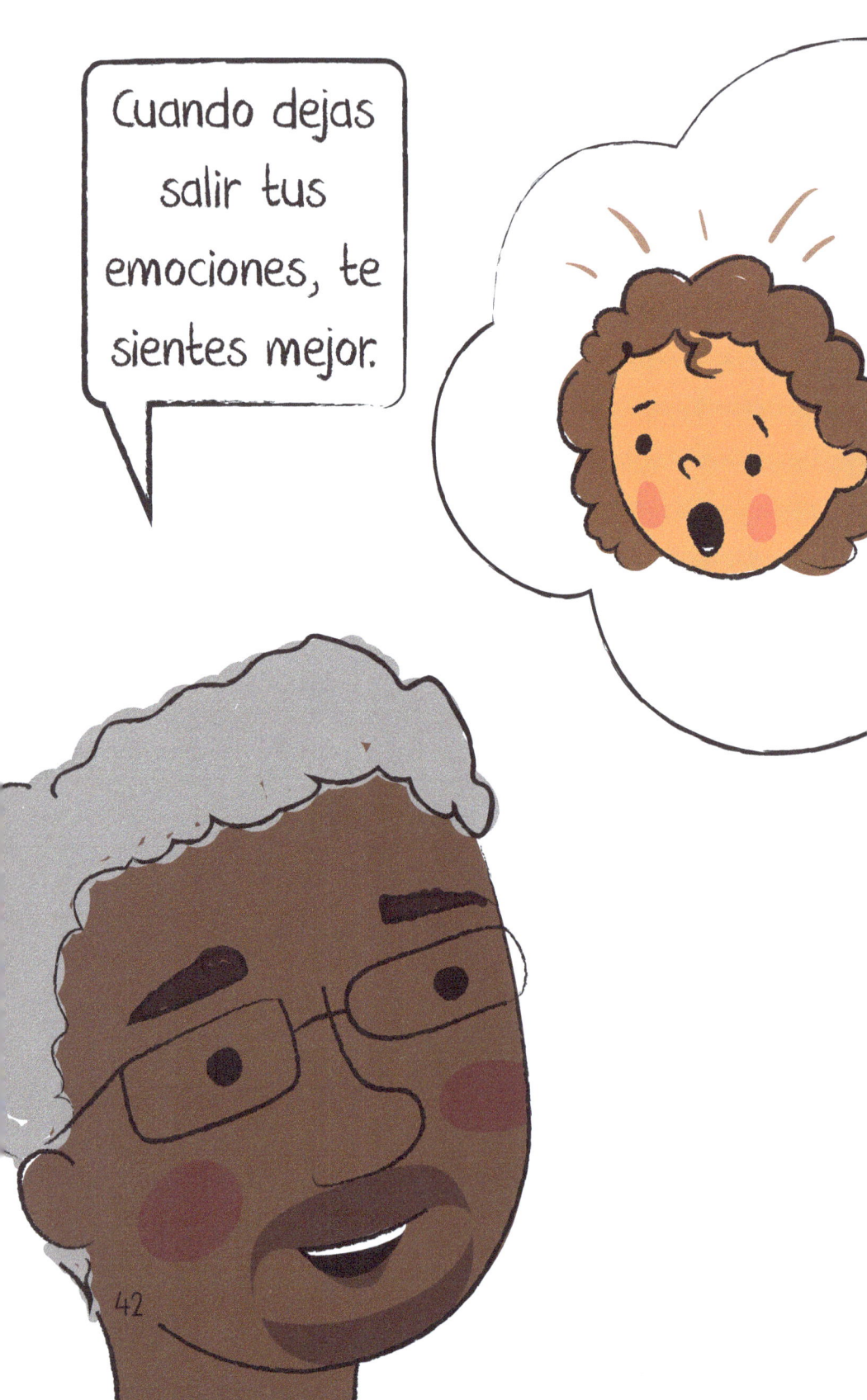

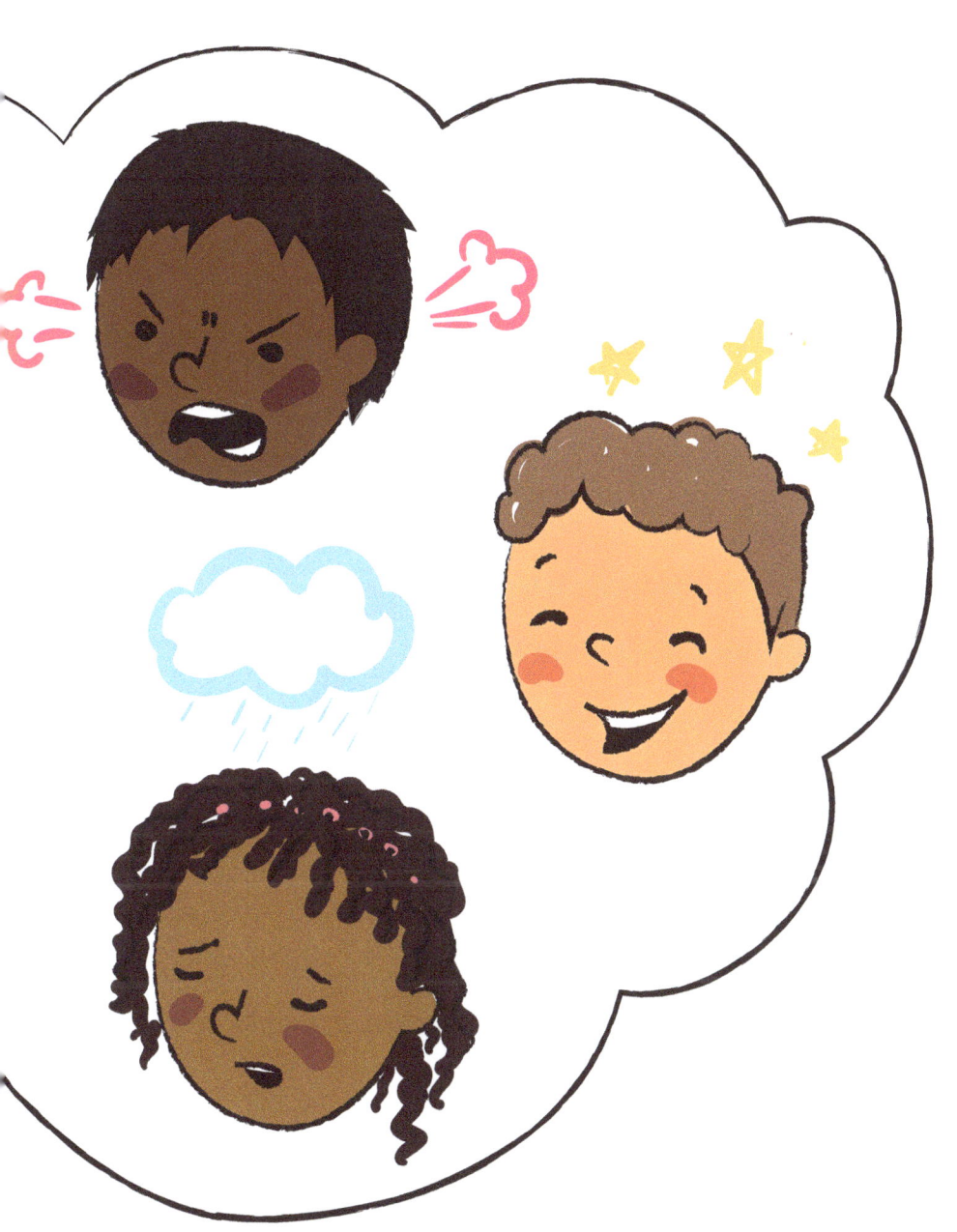

When you let your emotions out, you will feel better.

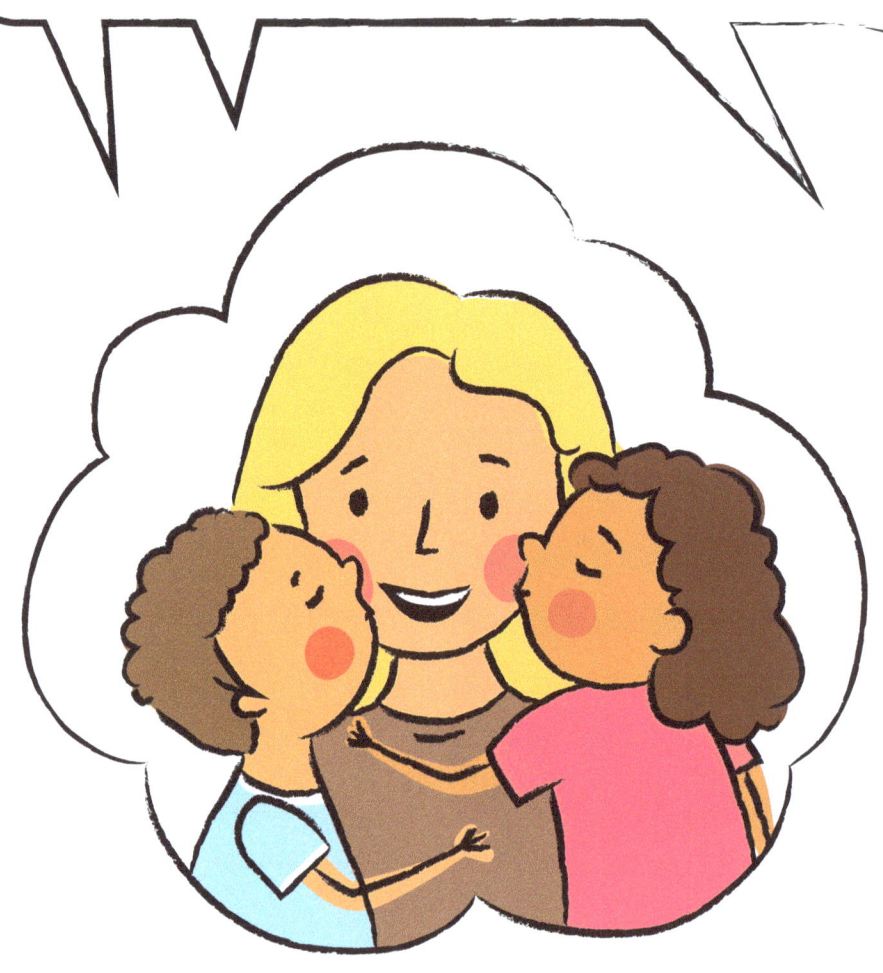

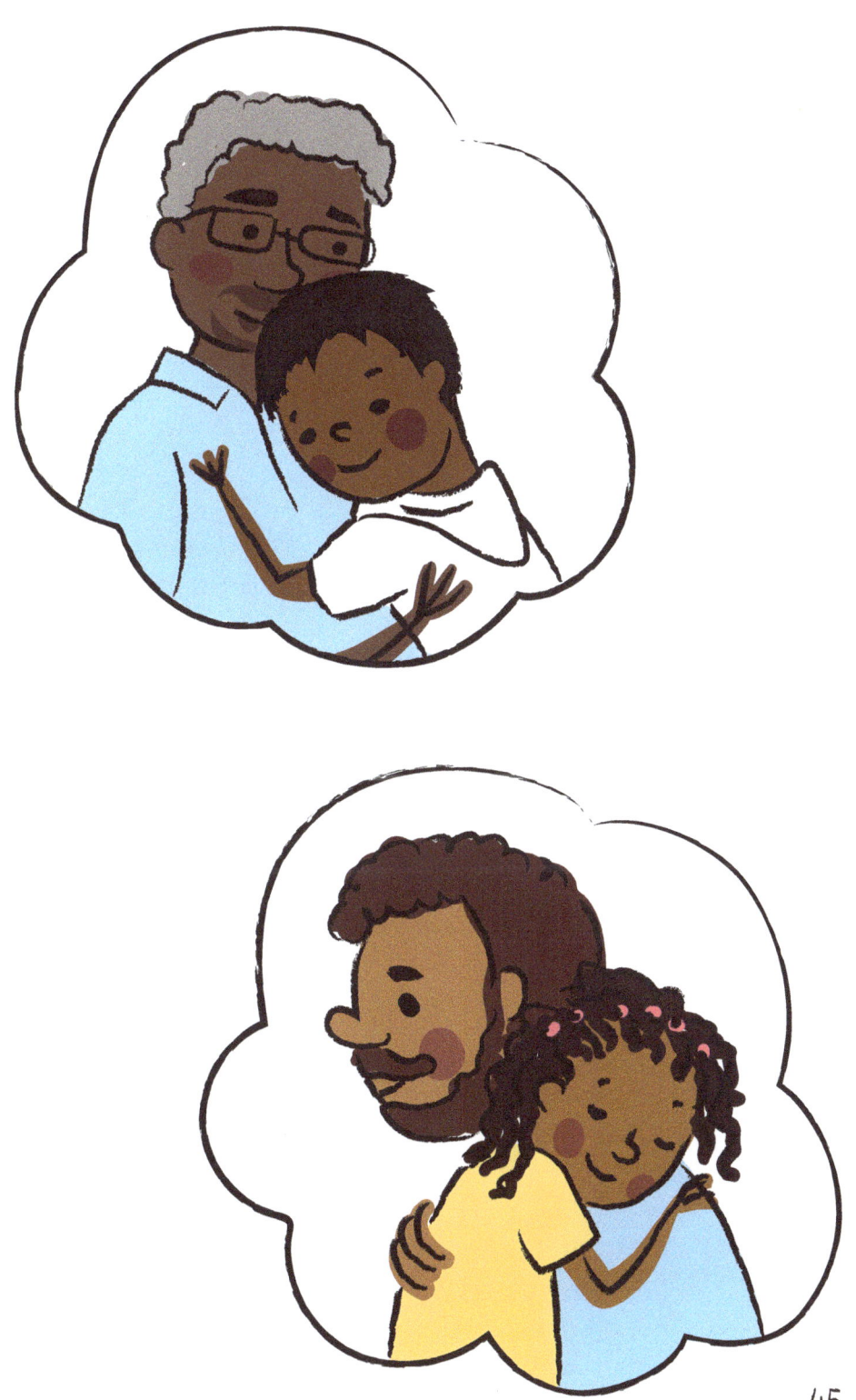

¡Expresa tus emociones!

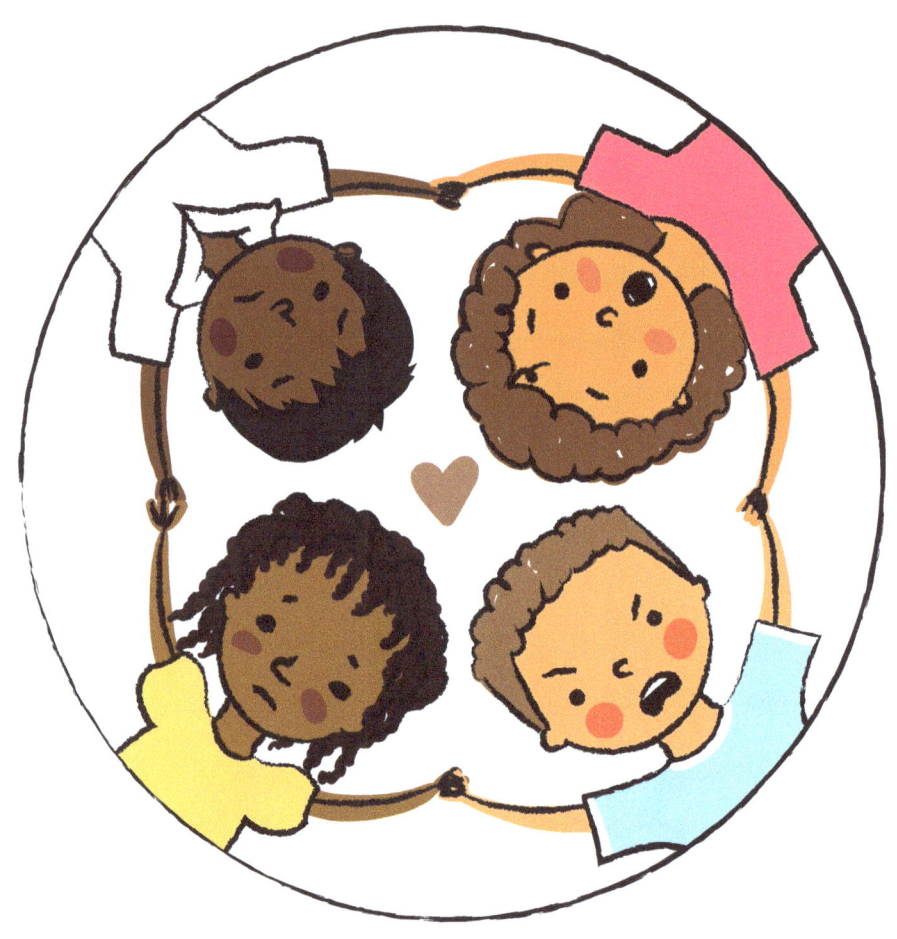

Let your emotions out!

TU VOCABULARIO BILINGÜE
YOUR BILINGUAL VOCABULARY

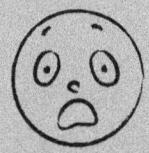
asustado
scared

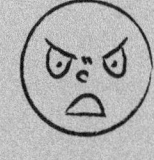
enfadado
angry

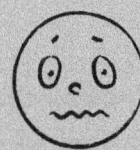
preocupado
worried

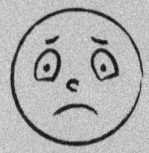
triste
sad

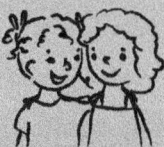
amigos
friends

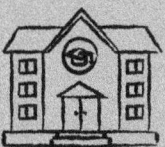
escuela
school

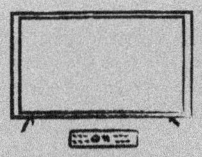
tele
TV

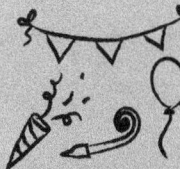
fiesta
party

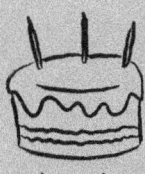
tarta
cake

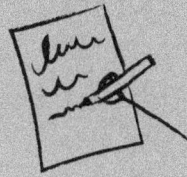
escribir
write

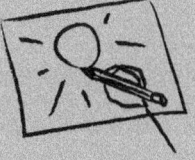
dibujar
draw

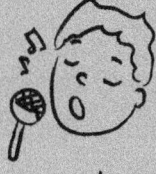
cantar
sing

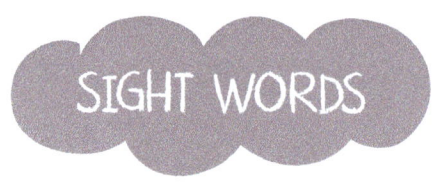

YOUNG & BILINGUAL ™ SIGHT WORDS TIPS

Sight words are words that don't follow the rules of spelling or syllable decoding. Children are taught as pre-readers to memorize sight words as a whole, by sight, so that they can recognize them immediately (within a few seconds). The goal is to read sight words without having to use decoding skills.

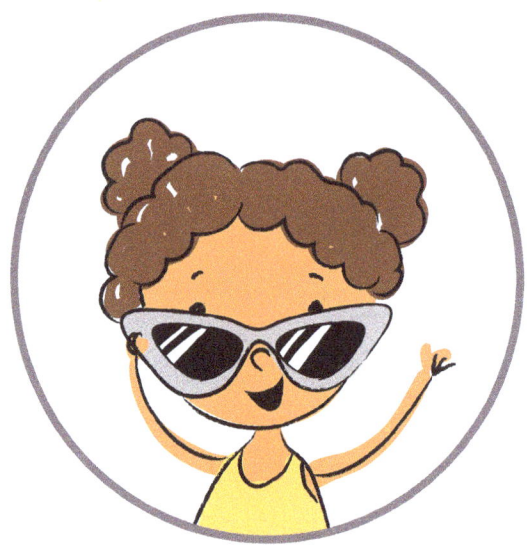

CONSEJOS PARA PALABRAS VISUALES DE YOUNG & BILINGUAL ™

Las palabras visuales son palabras que no siguen las reglas de ortografía o decodificación de sílabas. A los niños se les enseña como prelectores a memorizar las palabras visuales en su conjunto, a simple vista, para que puedan reconocerlas de inmediato (en unos segundos). El objetivo es leer palabras visuales sin tener que usar habilidades de decodificación.

SIGHT WORDS FROM THE BOOK

position
on in by out

action
get let

pronouns
you I my their them we your my us it

basic
why and that not with this to so many of the still a who but next all when other now no much are will am did be is was can have

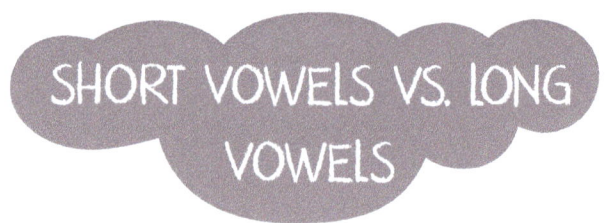

SHORT VOWELS VS. LONG VOWELS

YOUNG & BILINGUAL ™ QUICK PRONUNCIATION TIPS

- 'long vowel' is the term used to refer to vowel sounds whose pronunciation is the same as its letter name. The five vowels of the English language are 'a', 'e', 'i', 'o', 'u'.
- Each letter has a corresponding short vowel sound.
- When a word has two vowels, usually, the first vowel is pronounced as a long vowel and the second vowel is silent.

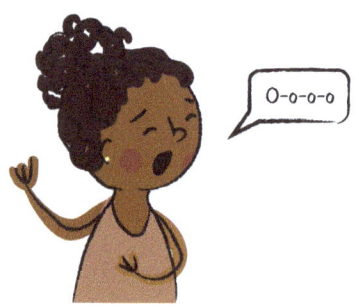

CONSEJOS DE PRONUNCIACIÓN DE YOUNG & BILINGUAL ™

- 'Vocal larga' es el término utilizado para referirse a los sonidos de las vocales cuya pronunciación es la misma que el nombre de su letra. Las cinco vocales del idioma inglés son ('a,' 'e,' 'i,' 'o,' y 'u').
- Cada letra tiene un sonido de vocal corta correspondiente.
- Cuando una palabra tiene dos vocales, por lo general, la primera vocal se pronuncia como una vocal larga y la segunda vocal es silenciosa.

LONG VOWELS		SHORT VOWELS
I life	**I**	will missed
afraid birthday	**A**	sad daddy
see year	**E**	never upset
Pipo so	**O**	mommy not
you graduate	**U**	cut grateful

BILINGUAL ENGLISH-SPANISH BOOKS

You will find level 1, 2, 3 and 4 books to suit the needs of your child or students!

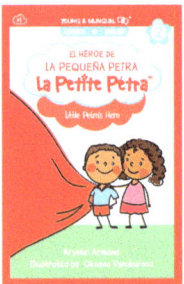 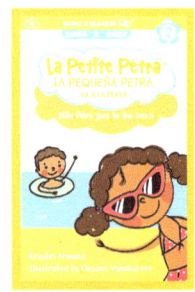 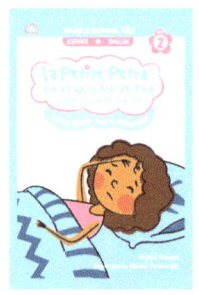 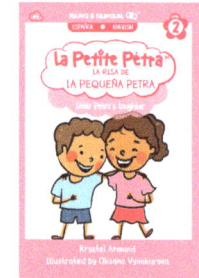

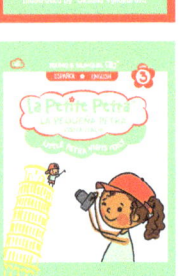 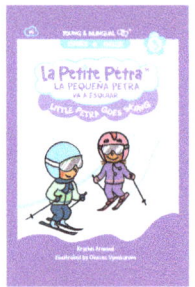 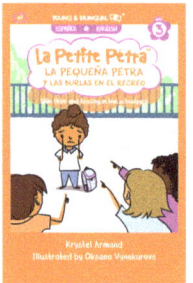 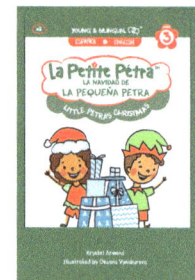

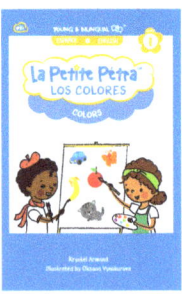 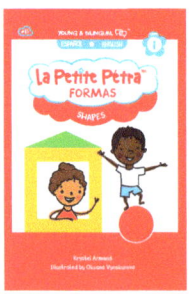 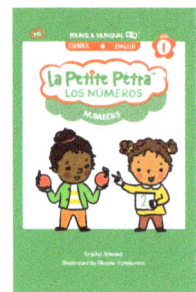 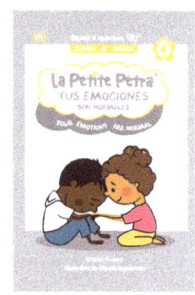

LIBROS BILINGÜES INGLÉS-ESPAÑOL

Encontrarás libros de los niveles 1,2,3 y 4 que se adaptarán a las necesidades de tus hijos o estudiantes.

Our bilingual book series also includes books in Creole-English, Portuguese-English and French-English, and come with a lot of additional materials! Download our catalog at www.lapetitepetra.com to view all our titles today!

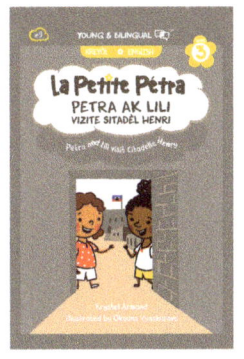
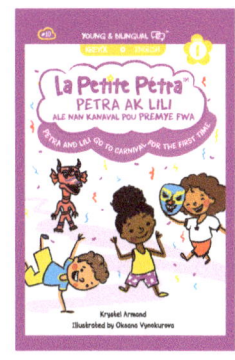
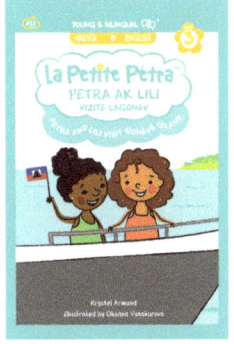
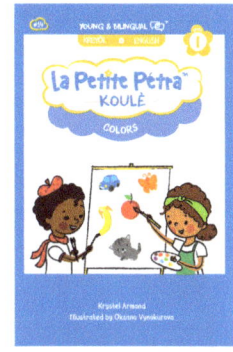

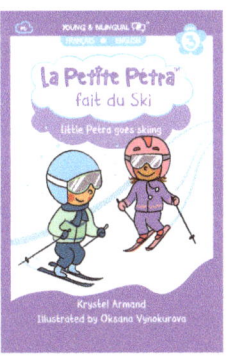
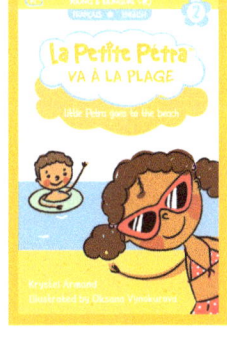
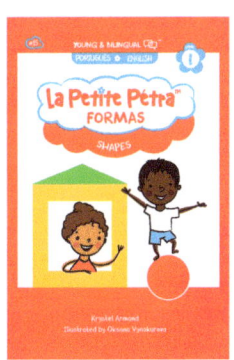
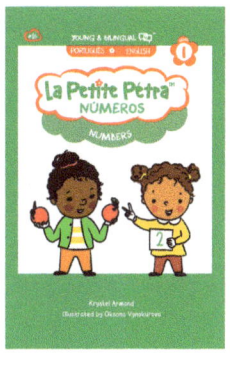

Nuestra serie de libros bilingües también incluye libros en criollo-inglés, portugués-inglés y francés-inglés, ¡y vienen con un montón de materiales adicionales! ¡Descarga nuestro catálogo en www.lapetitepetra.com para ver todos nuestros títulos hoy mismo!

www.ingramcontent.com/pod-product-compliance
Lightning Source LLC
Chambersburg PA
CBHW041132110526
44592CB00020B/2784